T0405816

Deep Pelvic Endometriosis

Paola De Nardi · Stefano Ferrari

Deep Pelvic Endometriosis

A Multidisciplinary Approach

With the contribution of
Elaine Denny

Foreword by
Massimo Candiani

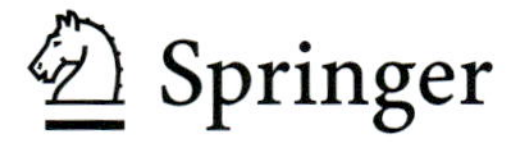

Springer

Authors
Paola De Nardi
Department of Surgery
San Raffaele Scientific Institute
Milan, Italy

Stefano Ferrari
Department of Obstetrics and Gynaecology
San Raffaele Scientific Institute
Milan, Italy

With the contribution of:
Elaine Denny
Professor of Health Sociology
Faculty of Health
Birmingham City University
Birmingham, UK

ISBN 978-88-470-1865-5 e-ISBN 978-88-470-1866-2

DOI 10.1007/978-88-470-1866-2

Springer Milan Dordrecht Heidelberg London New York

Library of Congress Control Number: 2010939273

9 8 7 6 5 4 3 2 1

Cover design: Ikona s.r.l., Milan, Italy

Typesetting: Graphostudio, Milan, Italy
Printing and binding: Arti Grafiche Nidasio, Assago (MI), Italy
Printed in Italy

Springer-Verlag Italia S.r.l. – Via Decembrio 28 – I-20137 Milan
Springer is a part of Springer Science+Business Media (www.springer.com)

Foreword

Deep endometriosis was identified by Cullen at the beginning of the last century, as a nodular lesion that is able to invade the rectovaginal space, the uterine ligaments, the wall of the bowel, and the ovary. Indeed, Cullen made a great contribution to progress in the field of defining and describing deeply invasive lesions, while Sampson was the first to describe superficial lesions with little or no associated smooth muscle metaplasia, minor symptoms, and fewer structural changes in the pelvis. Deep infiltrating endometriosis (DIE) is currently a specific entity defined by the presence of an endometriotic lesion that extends more than 5 mm below the peritoneum and includes infiltrative forms that involve vital structures such as the bowel, ureters, and bladder.

Some aspects of this condition have yet to be elucidated. The pathogenesis of this disorder has long been a source of debate, since some authors support its origin from previous Müllerian remnants, while others suggest that it derives from retrograde menstruation. In recent years, the potential peculiarity of the etiopathogenesis of DIE has received much attention from histologic, molecular, and clinical points of view. Another open problem is represented by the potential progression of the disease. There is actually no clear evidence that all deep nodules will necessarily progress to or acquire a destructive invasive phenotype. On the other hand, DIE is the only macroscopic lesion type where the relationship with pain symptoms appears to be well understood. The painful symptoms connected with DIE present particular characteristics that distinguish them from the painful symptoms of other etiology, as they are related to the involvement of the DIE implants in specific anatomical locations (severe dyspareunia) or organs (functional urinary tract signs and bowel signs). Infiltration of the pelvic nerves by the lesions explains the parallel between their anatomical location and the pain experienced by the patient. This aspect probably accounts for the fact that great attention has recently been focused on this condition, as it represents one of the main clinical problems affecting patients' health-related quality of life and can be devastating when vital organs are involved. Furthermore, DIE and surgery for this process are associated with increased complications. Preoperative recognition of DIE is highly desirable, since medical suppression before surgical intervention is likely to result in fewer complications and less operative difficulty.

This book was written in an attempt to clarify the various aspects of this problematic disease. The time has come to use a multidisciplinary approach to address this physically and psychologically distressing affliction, as has been proposed within the context of the overall clinical management of endometriosis. The book will be a valuable tool for gynecologists who want to update and increase the depth of their knowledge of urological and intestinal surgery, in order to improve their skills in daily practice. It is also directed to other specialists, urologists, and general surgeons, who are often involved in the diagnosis and treatment of this condition, even though it is not the exact focus of their expertise.

Milan, October 2010

Massimo Candiani
Director
Department of Obstetrics and Gynaecology
San Raffaele Scientific Institute
Milan, Italy

Contents

Abbreviations and Acronyms

3DUS	three-dimensional ultrasonography
AFS	American Fertility Association
COX-2	cyclo-oxygenase-2
CT	computerized tomography
DCBE	double-contrast barium enema
DIE	deeply infiltrating endometriosis
DPI	deep pelvic infiltration
EUS	endoscopic transrectal ultrasonography
GnRH	gonadotropin-releasing hormone
GP	general practitioner
HT	hormonal therapy
IBS	irritable bowel syndrome
IVP	intravenous pyelography
LUNA	laparoscopic uterosacral nerve ablation
MRI	magnetic resonance imaging
NPV	negative predictive value
PC	partial cystectomy
PN	presacral neurectomy
PPV	positive predictive value
r-AFS	revised American Fertility Association (classification)
RCT	randomized controlled trial
RWC-TVS	rectal water-contrast transvaginal sonography
ST	surgical therapy
TNF-α	tumor necrosis factor-α
TUR	transurethral resection
TVS	transvaginal sonography
UE	ureteral endometriosis
UR	ureteroscopy
US	ultrasonography

Introduction

1

P. De Nardi, S. Ferrari

Abstract Endometriosis, defined as the presence of endometrial gland tissue and stroma outside the uterus, is a common disease with an estimated prevalence of 10% in women of reproductive age. Deep pelvic endometriosis is a specific entity defined by endometriotic lesions extending more than 5 mm under the peritoneum, usually located in the pouch of Douglas and in the connective tissue of the rectovaginal septum, that may involve the uterosacral ligaments, the rectum or the rectosigmoid junction, and the urinary tract.

Several theories have been proposed for the pathogenesis of deep pelvic endometriosis, namely the implantation of regurgitated endometrium, the theory of Müllerian or coelomic remnants metaplasia, the direct transplantation theory, and the theory of dissemination through the lymphatic and blood vessels.

The most-used classification-system for endometriosis is currently The American Fertility Society revised (r-AFS) classification, but other systems have been proposed by Konincks and Martin, Martin and Butt, Adamyan, and, more recently, by Chapron. Unfortunately, no system is universally shared.

Keywords r-ASF • Peritoneum • Cul-de-sac • Pouch of Douglas

P. De Nardi (✉)
Department of Surgery, San Raffaele Scientific Institute, Milan, Italy

1.1 Definition, Prevalence, and Epidemiology

Endometriosis is defined as the presence of endometrial glands and stroma outside the endometrial cavity and uterine musculature. These ectopic endometrial implants are usually located in the pelvis, but can occur nearly anywhere in the body.

The prevalence of endometriosis in specific categories of patients has been reported, but the prevalence in the general population is not known [1–3].

The most important risk factors for endometriosis are nulliparity, early menarche, polymenorrhea, and hypermenorrhea [4]. Endometriosis also appears to be associated with a taller, thinner body habitus and lower body mass index [5]. The prevalence appears to be higher in Caucasian than in Black or Asian populations [3].

The growth and maintenance of endometriotic implants are influenced by ovarian steroids. As a result, endometriosis occurs during the active reproductive period: in women aged 25 to 35 years [5, 6]. They are uncommon in pre- or post-menarchal girls [7–9], and rare in postmenopausal women who are not taking hormones.

1.2 Pathogenesis

Several theories relating to the pathogenesis of endometriosis have been put forward since its first description by von Rokitansky in 1860 [10–12].

- The “implantation” theory proposes that endometrial tissue from the uterus is shed during menstruation and transported through the fallopian tubes (retrograde menstruation), thereby gaining access to and implanting on pelvic structures [13].
- The second theory is that of “metaplasia” (Meyer 1919) [14] – either coelomic (peritoneal) metaplasia (Gruenwald 1942) [15] or Müllerian remnants metaplasia (Donnez 1995) [16]. The first hypothesis is based upon embryologic studies demonstrating that all pelvic organs, including the endometrium, are derived from cells lining the coelomic cavity. The other one is based on the metaplastic potential of the Müllerian cells present in the rectovaginal septum.
- The direct transplantation theory is the probable explanation for

endometriosis that develops in episiotomy, cesarean section, and other scars after surgery.

- Endometriosis in locations outside the pelvis is explained by dissemination of endometrial cells or tissue through the lymphatic and blood vessels.

1.2.1 Retrograde Menstruation

Numerous studies have demonstrated that reflux of endometrial cells into the peritoneal cavity is a very common physiologic condition that occurs during normal menstruation in most women with patent tubes [17, 18]. The viability of endometrial cells has been demonstrated by culture of the menstrual effluent or peritoneal fluid [19, 20]. Therefore, anatomic alterations of the pelvis that increase tubal reflux of menstrual endometrium should increase a woman's chance of developing endometriosis.

Evidence supporting this hypothesis is derived from the observation that the incidence of endometriosis is increased in girls with genital tract obstructions that prevent expulsion of menses into the vagina and therefore increase the likelihood of tubal reflux [21]. The development of endometriosis should also be related to additional factors, such as the amount of endometrial tissue reaching the peritoneal cavity and/or the capacity to eliminate the refluxed menstrual debris.

There are two main possibilities that explain endometrioma formation. The first mechanism is due to superficial implantation of regurgitated endometrial cells and subsequent adhesion between the gonad and the peritoneum of the ovarian fossa, and the broad ligament and invagination of the cortex [22]. The second possibility is the colonization of a functional cyst by regurgitated endometrium, as first hypothesized by Sampson [22]. Vercellini et al recently supported this theory. They sonographically observed a progression from a hemorrhagic corpus luteum to an endometrioma. Therefore, the typical "chocolate fluid" entrapped in the cyst may originate from bleeding of corpora lutea. This would explain why the volume of endometriotic cysts may increase suddenly, as well as why the wall may be devoid of endometrial lining [23].

1.2.2 Altered Immunity

In women who develop endometriosis, the endometrial cells escape being cleared by the immune response, attach to peritoneal mesothelial cells, and then invade into the extracellular matrix, where they proliferate into macroscopic disease.

Several studies have demonstrated an altered humoral and cell-mediated immunity in patients developing endometriosis:

- deficient cellular immunity may result in an inability to recognize the presence of endometrial tissue in abnormal locations [24];
- natural killer cell activity may be reduced, resulting in decreased cytotoxicity to autologous endometrium [25];
- there is an increased concentration of leukocytes and macrophages in the peritoneal cavity and in ectopic endometrium [26, 27]. These cells secrete cytokines (for example, interleukin-1, 6, and 8, tumor necrosis factors, RANTES) and growth factors into the peritoneal fluid of women with endometriosis [28].

Furthermore, an association of endometriosis with higher rates of autoimmune inflammatory diseases, hypothyroidism, fibromyalgia, chronic fatigue syndrome, allergies, and asthma, has been found [29].

1.2.3 Genetic Factors

Genetic factors probably influence an individual's susceptibility to endometriosis [30–32]. The possibility of a familial tendency for endometriosis has been recognized for several decades. Concordance in twins has also been observed [30].

1.2.4 Gross and Microscopic Pathology

The appearance and size of the implants are quite variable. Areas of peritoneal endometriosis appear as raised flame-like patches, whitish opacifications, yellow-brown discoloration, translucent blebs, or reddish or reddish-blue irregularly shaped islands. The peritoneal surface may be scarred or puckered.

Endometriosis of the ovary may present as superficial implants, or as pelvic masses comprising cyst-like structures (endometriomas) that contain blood, fluid, and menstrual debris.

The microscopic appearance of endometriotic tissue is similar to that of

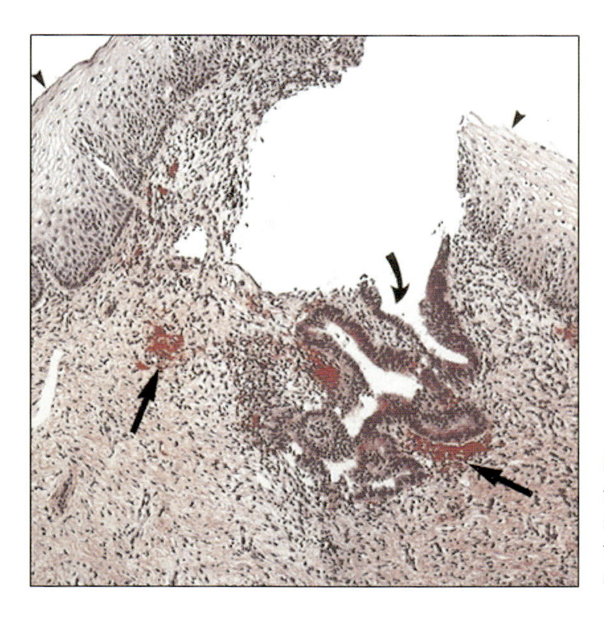

Fig. 1.1 Light micrograph of peritoneal endometriotic implant shows endometrial glandular epithelium (*arrow*) and surrounding stroma

endometrium in the uterine cavity; the two major components of both are endometrial glands and stroma (Fig. 1.1). Unlike endometrium, however, endometriotic implants often contain fibrous tissue, blood, and cysts.

1.2.5 Link to Cancer

Epidemiological evidence from most large cohort studies suggests that endometriosis is an independent risk factor for epithelial ovarian cancer. One review including several of these studies found the prevalence of endometriosis in serous, mucinous, clear-cell, and endometrioid ovarian carcinoma was 4.5%, 1.4%, 35.9%, and 19.0%, respectively, and the risk of malignant transformation of ovarian endometriosis was estimated to be 2.5% [33].

1.3 Deep Endometriosis

As noted before, endometriosis is a very controversial disease. There are three types of endometriosis: superficial endometriosis, ovarian endometrioma, and deeply infiltrating endometriosis (DIE). Recently, great attention has been focused on deep endometriosis. In the late 1980s, CO_2-laser-excision techniques led to the observation that some typical lesions infiltrate deep into the subperitoneal stroma [34, 35]. DIE is a specific entity defined by the presence of an endometriotic lesion extending more than 5 mm underneath the peritoneum [35], including the infiltrative forms that involve vital structures, such as the bowel, ureters, and bladder, as well as forms such as many rectovaginal lesions [36]. The choice of 5 mm was made in light of epidemiologic observation [37]. Morphologically, superficial endometriosis is an active disease in only about 50% of lesions [34]. Lesions infiltrating only a few millimeters (mostly typical lesions) frequently have a burnt-out aspect, whereas lesions infiltrating deeper than 5 mm are morphologically the most active lesions. Clinical observations suggest that in the majority of women the endometriotic lesion infiltrates only superficially, and becomes inactive; however, when lesions infiltrate deeper than 5 mm, the disease becomes more active and aggressive and develops into a much deeper lesion [37]. The most severe form of deep endometriosis is characterized by extensive and painful nodularities of the pouch of Douglas.

Some authors have suggested that deep endometriosis may have different etiopathologic mechanisms from those of pelvic and ovarian endometriosis [38, 39].

Deep lesions of the posterior cul-de-sac correspond to adenomyotic nodule originating from metaplasia of Müllerian remnants located in the rectovaginal septum, thus constituting a different entity from peritoneal endometriosis [38]. On the other hand, it has been suggested that peritoneal endometriosis originates from implantation of regurgitated endometrium. Ovarian endometriosis is still a source of controversy: there is still contradiction between theories of implantation and metaplasia. This hypothesis is based upon the typical histological aspect of the different localization and type.

In fact, endometriotic rectovaginal nodules show a similar histological aspect to adenomyotic nodules: they appear as an isolated aggregate of smooth muscle, endometrial glands, and usually endometrial stroma [40–42]. Invasion of the smooth muscle by active glandular epithelium without stroma proves that stroma is not necessary for invasion, and that the deep posterior nodule is different from peritoneal endometriosis, in which epithelial glands are surrounded systematically by endometrial-type stroma.

Adenomyosis exhibits an altered response to ovarian hormones: proliferative glands and stroma are observed in the first half of the menstrual cycle, but this is not always followed by secretory changes, which may be absent or incomplete during the second half of the menstrual cycle. These histological observations are possible even in endometriotic rectovaginal nodules (Fig. 1.2).

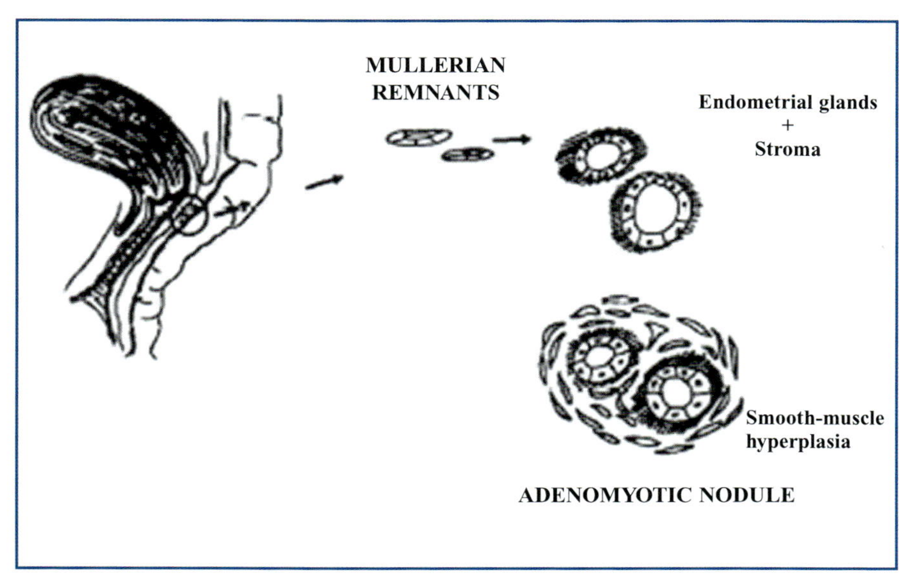

Fig. 1.2 Hypothesis of histogenesis of rectovaginal endometriosis. Reproduced from [38], with permission

Some authors, on the other hand, suggest the hypothesis that the three forms of endometriosis (DIE, peritoneal, and ovarian) share a single pathogenesis, namely implantation of regurgitated endometrium [43–49]. This is supported by an epidemiological study demonstrating that women with deep, pelvic, and ovarian endometriosis have a similar epidemiological profile. They share both protective and risk factors. DIE could be the most severe manifestation of peritoneal disease [48].

Considering the high prevalence of other forms of endometriosis in patients with deep endometriosis, a prevalence that is different from that expected in the general population, a similar pathogenetic mechanism leading to the different forms of disease can be considered [46].

The pathogenetic pathway leading to anatomic distortion begins with superficial implantation of endometrial cells, which triggers a strong inflammatory stimulus. The pelvic structures adhere to the site of ectopic implants, trying to circumscribe the irritating lesion, and to exclude it from the peritoneal environment. The ensuing scar retraction may cause duplication and invagination of adjacent surfaces, contributing to engulfing endometrial foci. The process may drag various structures around endometriotic implants with their final encirclement. When the ovary is involved, an endometriotic cyst may develop [50], whereas duplication of anterior cul-de-sac peritoneum initiates bladder detrusor endometriosis [51]. When the process involves the sigmoid or, more rarely, the cecum, a distinct, large, and hard nodule forms. This lesion most often consists of duplicated and invaginated intestinal wall with very limited endometriotic tissue.

Another observation in favor of the theory of regurgitation concerns the anatomical distribution of pelvic DIE. DIE lesions present a double asymmetry [49]: they are more frequently observed in the posterior compartment and most often located in the left side. With the patient standing erect, because of gravity, menstrual blood reflux accumulates in the pouch of Douglas. This also explains why pelvic DIE lesions are more frequently observed than high-abdominal DIE, and why intestinal DIE lesions are preferentially located on the rectum and rectosigmoid junction.

The anatomical differences between the left and right hemipelvis, because of the presence of the sigmoid colon on the left side, explain the prevalence of left-located lesions. The close anatomical relationship between the sigmoid colon and the left adnexa forms an isolated site, which results in an anatomical situation that could encourage adhesions and growth of regurgitated endometrial cells [43, 52–54].

The flow of peritoneal fluid, as well as regurgitated endometrial cells, also plays a part in DIE pathogenesis. Meyers [55] demonstrated that intraperitoneal fluid continually circulates through the abdomen in a clockwise direction, due to bowel peristalsis and changes in hydrostatic pressure because of movement of the diaphragm.

The vast majority of the fibrotic plaques of the posterior cul-de-sac are located in the retrocervical area [56–58], and the detrusor nodules are usually found adhering to the uterine body. It has been suggested that DIE originates from metaplasia of Müllerian remnants located in the rectovaginal and vescicovaginal septa. Otherwise these septa may not be the real site of deep nodular endometriosis, because, based on normal anatomy, the rectovaginal septum is located caudally with respect to the posterior vaginal fornix, and the vescicovaginal septum, by definition, does not extend beyond the cervix [59].

If the theory of Müllerian remnants metaplasia were true, the anatomy of the pouch of Douglas should be similar in women with and without DIE, because if these lesions originate in the rectovaginal septum, they should be located extraperitoneally. On the other hand, if deep foci were a manifestation of intraperitoneal disease, the pouch of Douglas should be partially or completely obliterated in affected women.

The mean depth of the rectovaginal pouch in normal women, as measured from the upper border of the uterosacral ligaments to its base, has been demonstrated to be slightly over 5 cm, regardless of parity or prolapse

[60, 61]. Patients with deep endometriotic lesions, but not women with other forms of endometriosis or other pathology, have about one-third reduction in the depth of the cul-de-sac. Partial obliteration by the anterior rectal wall, subsequent to inflammatory process due to peritoneal implantation of regurgitated endometrial cells, is the cause of this apparent reduction and may give the false impression that nodules are subperitoneal [36].

Although the previous arguments support a common pathogenetic mechanism for the different forms of endometriosis, they do not clarify why, from a histological point of view, deep endometriotic nodules, but not the other forms of the disease, resemble adenomyosis. In this regard, it has to be noted that Anaf et al [62], using immunochemical techniques with a monoclonal antibody against muscle-specific actin, recently demonstrated that a smooth muscle component is in fact present in all types of endometriotic lesions. On the other hand, they failed to observe this component in disease-free peritoneum. These authors thus hypothesize that the smooth muscle component may result from the totipotential capacity of the pelvic and lower abdomen mesothelium to differentiate. In other words, the implanted endometrium may cause a metaplastic response in the underlying tissue. This metaplastic response might differ from one location to the other, thus explaining histological differences among the various forms of endometriosis [46].

1.4 Classification

A valid and reliable classification must possess some characteristics: easy comprehension and reproducibility of the severity of the condition, leading to therapeutic strategies, and identification of the prognosis. A staging system must comprehend the natural history of the disease, its local invasiveness, and functional, as well as organic consequences. This scheme must consider sequential steps of severity, with a specific link with the outcome of interest. There are different classifications of deep endometriosis in the literature, but more studies are needed to demonstrate that the proposed classifications meet the above criteria.

Currently, the most used classification system for endometriosis is The American Fertility Society revised (r-AFS) classification. The original and revised AFS classifications are unique because they provide a standardized form for recording pathologic findings, and because they assign scalar values to disease status in an effort to predict the probability of pregnancy following treatment [63, 64].

The scoring system of the r-AFS is directed at the variability in assessing ovarian endometriosis and cul-de-sac obliteration.

To improve the accuracy of the scoring system, ovarian endometriotic cyst should be confirmed by histology or by the presence of the following features: (1) cyst diameter <12 cm; (2) adhesion to the pelvic side wall and/or broad ligament; (3) endometriosis on surface of ovary; and (4) tarry, thick, chocolate-coloured fluid content [65].

Cul-de-sac obliteration should be considered partial if endometriosis or adhesions have obliterated part of the cul-de-sac, but some normal peritoneum is visible below the uterosacral ligaments. Complete obliteration of the cul-de-sac exists when no peritoneum is visible below the uterosacral ligaments. The morphology of peritoneal and ovarian implants should be categorized as red (red, red-pink, and clear lesions), white (white, yellow-brown, and peritoneal defects), and black (black and blue lesions) [66]. The percentage of surface involvement of each implant type should be documented (Fig. 1.3).

It seems easy to consider DIE as stage IV of the r-AFS classification. However, this scheme was devised mainly with the object of stratifying patients according to their reproductive prognosis. This is because great value is attributed to ovarian endometriomas in the r-AFS classification. A finding of a bilateral 4 cm ovarian cyst is sufficient to reach a point score indicating severe or fourth-stage endometriosis, according to the patient's reproductive outcome. On the other hand, this apparently advanced stage could be easily improved by a simple surgical approach, whereas a second-stage endometriosis could represent a more difficult situation for the surgeon if the total score is obtained by considering the extent of adherences, which often require a laparotomic approach.

Konincks and Martin [39, 67] were the first to define deep endometriosis. They distinguished posterior cul-de-sac and rectovaginal lesions in three different subgroups: type I, a conically shaped lesion derived from infiltration; type II, a deeply located lesion, surrounded by extensive bowel retraction and adhesions; and type III, the most severe form, one or more spherical nodules located in the rectovaginal septum with the largest dimension under the peritoneum, which appears as a small typical lesion or sometimes even a normal peritoneum overlying an induration.

Another classification has been presented by Adamyan [68], who classified specifically retrocervical endometriosis into four stages according to the extent of disease in the retrocervical area: in stage I, endometriotic lesions are confined to rectovaginal cellular tissue in the area of the vaginal vault; stage II exists when endometriotic tissue invades the cervix and penetrates the vaginal wall, causing fibrosis and small cyst formation; in stage III, lesions spread into the uterosacral ligaments and the rectal serosa. The last

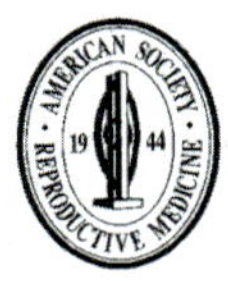

AMERICAN SOCIETY FOR REPRODUCTIVE MEDICINE
REVISED CLASSIFICATION OF ENDOMETRIOSIS

Patient's Name ______ Date ______

Stage I (Minimal) - 1-5
Stage II (Mild) - 6-15
Stage III (Moderate) - 16-40
Stage IV (Severe) - >40
Total ______

Laparoscopy ______ Laparotomy ______ Photography ______
Recommended Treatment ______

Prognosis ______

	ENDOMETRIOSIS	<1cm	1-3cm	>3cm
PERITONEUM	Superficial	1	2	4
	Deep	2	4	6
OVARY	R Superficial	1	2	4
	Deep	4	16	20
	L Superficial	1	2	4
	Deep	4	16	20

POSTERIOR CULDESAC OBLITERATION	Partial	Complete
	4	40

	ADHESIONS	<1/3 Enclosure	1/3-2/3 Enclosure	>2/3 Enclosure
OVARY	R Filmy	1	2	4
	Dense	4	8	16
	L Filmy	1	2	4
	Dense	4	8	16
TUBE	R Filmy	1	2	4
	Dense	4*	8*	16
	L Filmy	1	2	4
	Dense	4*	8*	16

***If the fimbriated end of the fallopian tube is completely enclosed, change the point assignment to 16.**

Denote appearance of superficial implant types as red [(R), red, red-pink, flamelike, vesicular blobs, clear vesicles], white [(W), opacifications, peritoneal defects, yellow-brown], or black [(B) black, hemosiderin deposits, blue]. Denote percent of total described as R___%, W___% and B___%. Total should equal 100%.

Additional Endometriosis: ______

Associated Pathology: ______

To Be Used with Normal Tubes and Ovaries

L R

To Be Used with Abnormal Tubes and/or Ovaries

L R

Fig. 1.3 The revised American Fertility Association classification of endometriosis. Reproduced from [64], with permission

and most severe stage, IV, exists when the rectal wall, rectosigmoid zone, and retro-uterine peritoneum are completely involved, and the recto-uterine pouch is totally obliterated [68].

Martin and Batt [56] differentiated between retrocervical, rectovaginal pouch, and rectovaginal septum endometriosis. This differentiation is important because deep endometriosis infiltrating from the peritoneum to the vagina can be treated with a relatively easy outpatient procedure when the rectum is not involved. On the other hand, rectovaginal endometriosis, particularly with involvement of the rectovaginal septum, requires more complex surgery and is associated with a higher rate of complications. Retrocervical endometriosis includes lesions in the anterior aspect of the pouch of Douglas, posterior vaginal fornix, and retroperitoneal area behind or beneath the cervix, with no rectal involvement. In rectovaginal endometriosis, the rectal and vaginal walls, as well as both vaginal and rectal aspects of the posterior cul-de-sac, are involved. Rectovaginal septum endometriosis refers to isolated, true subperitoneal lesions with no continuity with Douglas pouch lesions.

From a practical point of view, this classification is difficult to apply because of the frequent association that exists between the different DIE types and because true rectovaginal septum involvement is not easy to identify. Until now, these classifications place patients requiring different operative techniques into the same category. Therefore, another more recent classification takes the presence of both anterior and postero-uterine pouches into account, and suggests specific surgical procedures based on deep infil-

Table 1.1 Classification of deeply infiltrating endometriosis (DIE). Reproduced from [69], with permission

DIE classification	Operative procedure
A: Anterior DIE	
A1: Bladder	Laparoscopic partial cystectomy
P: Posterior DIE	
P1: Uterosacral ligaments	Laparoscopic resection of USL[a]
P2: Vagina	Laparoscopically assisted vaginal resection of DIE infiltrating the posterior fornix
P3: Intestine	
Solely intestinal location	
Without vaginal infiltration (V–)	Intestinal resection by laparoscopy or by laparotomy
With vaginal infiltration (V+)	Laparoscopically assisted vaginal intestinal resection or exeresis by laparotomy
Multiple intestinal location	Intestinal resection by laparotomy

[a]USL, uterosacral ligament

trating endometriosis stage [69]. Stages A (anterior pouch and bladder DIE) and P (posterior pouch DIE) are distinguished. The latter stage is divided into P1 substage (uterosacral ligaments lesions), P2 (vaginal lesions), and P3 (intestinal lesions). Substage P3 is further stratified into lesions with a solely intestinal location, without (V–) and with (V+) vaginal infiltration, and those with multiple intestinal locations (Table 1.1).

Clear and generally accepted classification for the study and treatment of endometriosis could improve patient care, permitting standard therapies and defining a realistic reproductive prognosis. Unfortunately, none of the classifications of DIE reported here are universally shared. More experience with the existing classification types must be provided to improve them and facilitate a choice of the most appropriate system for worldwide use.

Aknowledgments This chapter has been written with the collaboration of F. Di Puppo (Department of Obstetrics and Gynaecology, San Raffaele Scientific Institute, Milan, Italy), P. Persico (Department of Obstetrics and Gynaecology, San Raffaele Scientific Institute, Milan, Italy), and I. Tandoi (Department of Obstetrics and Gynaecology, San Raffaele Scientific Institute, Milan, Italy).

References

1. Sangi-Haghpeykar H, Poindexter AN 3rd. Epidemiology of endometriosis among parous women. Obstet Gynecol 1995;85:983–992
2. Chatman DL, Ward AB. Endometriosis in adolescents. J Reprod Med 1982;27:156–160
3. Missmer SA, Hankinson SE, Spiegelman D et al. Incidence of laparoscopically confirmed endometriosis by demographic, anthropometric, and lifestyle factors. Am J Epidemiol 2004;160:784–796
4. Missmer SA, Hankinson SE, Spiegelman D et al. Reproductive history and endometriosis among premenopausal women. Obstet Gynecol 2004;104:965–974
5. Hediger ML, Hartnett HJ, Louis GM. Association of endometriosis with body size and figure. Fertil Steril 2005;84:1366–1374
6. Olive DL, Schwartz LB. Endometriosis. N Engl J Med 1993;328:1759–1769
7. Laufer MR. Premenarcheal endometriosis without an associated obstructive anomaly: presentation, diagnosis, and treatment. Fertil Steril 2000;74:S15
8. Goldstein DP, deCholnoky C, Leventhal JM, Emans SJ. New insights into the old problem of chronic pelvic pain. J Pediatr Surg 1979;14:675–680
9. Yamamoto K, Mitsuhashi Y, Takaike T et al. Tubal endometriosis diagnosed within one month after menarche: a case report. Tohoku J Exp Med 1997;181:385–387
10. Schenken RS. Pathogenesis. In: Schenken RS (ed). Endometriosis: contemporary concepts in clinical management. JB Lippincott Company, Philadelphia, 1989, p 1
11. Bulun SE. Endometriosis. N Engl J Med 2009;360:268–279
12. von Rokitansky C. Ueber Uterusdrusen-Neubildung in Uterus and Ovarialsarcomen [Uterine gland proliferation in uterine and ovarian sarcomas]. Zeitschrift Gesellschaft für Aerzte zu Wien 1860;37:577

13. Sampson JA. Metastatic or embolic endometriosis, due to the menstrual dissemination of endometrial tissue into the venous circulation. Am J Pathol 1927;3:93–110
14. Meyer R. Uber den stand der frage der adenomyositis und adenomyoma in algemeinen und insbesondere uber adenomyositis und adenomyometritis sarcomatosa. Zentrlbl Gynäkol 1919;43:745–750
15. Gruenwald P. Origin of endometriosis from mesenchyme of the coelomic walls. Am J Obstet Gynecol 1942;44:470–474
16. Donnez J, Nisolle M, Casanas-Roux F et al. Rectovaginal septum, endometriosis or adenomyosis: laparoscopic management in a series of 231 patients. Hum Reprod 1995;10:630–635
17. Halme J, Hammond MG, Hulka JF et al. Retrograde menstruation in healthy women and in patients with endometriosis. Obstet Gynecol 1984;64:151–154
18. Liu DT, Hitchcock A. Endometriosis: its association with retrograde menstruation, dysmenorrhoea and tubal pathology. Br J Obstet Gynaecol 1986;93:859–862
19. Keettel WC, Stein RJ. The viability of the cast-off menstrual endometrium. Am J Obstet Gynecol 1951;61:440–442
20. Kruitwagen RF, Poels LG, Willemsen WN et al. Endometrial epithelial cells in peritoneal fluid during the early follicular phase. Fertil Steril 1991;55:297–303
21. Olive DL, Henderson DY. Endometriosis and mullerian anomalies. Obstet Gynecol 1987;69:412–415
22. Brosens IA, Puttemans P, Deprest J, Rombauts L. The endometriosis cycle and its derailments. Hum Reprod 1994;9:770–771
23. Vercellini P, Somigliana E, Vigano P et al. 'Blood On The Tracks' from corpora lutea to endometriomas. BJOG 2009;116:366–371
24. Steele RW, Dmowski WP, Marmer DJ. Immunologic aspects of human endometriosis. Am J Reprod Immunol 1984;6:33–36
25. Oosterlynck DJ, Cornillie FJ, Waer M et al. Women with endometriosis show a defect in natural killer activity resulting in a decreased cytotoxicity to autologous endometrium. Fertil Steril 1991;56:45–51
26. Dmowski WP, Gebel HM, Braun DP. The role of cell-mediated immunity in pathogenesis of endometriosis. Acta Obstet Gynecol Scand Suppl 1994;159:7–14
27. Witz CA. Interleukin-6: another piece of the endometriosis-cytokine puzzle. Fertil Steril 2000; 73:212–214
28. Bacci M, Capobianco A, Monno A et al. Macrophages are alternatively activated in patients with endometriosis and required for growth and vascularization of lesions in a mouse model of disease. Am J Pathol 2009;175:547–556
29. Sinaii N, Cleary SD, Ballweg ML et al. High rates of autoimmune and endocrine disorders, fibromyalgia, chronic fatigue syndrome and atopic diseases among women with endometriosis: a survey analysis. Hum Reprod 2002;17:2715–2724
30. Simpson JL, Bischoff F. Heritability and candidate genes for endometriosis. Reprod Biomed Online 2003;7:162–169
31. Campbell IG, Thomas EJ. Endometriosis: candidate genes. Hum Reprod Update 2001;7:15–20
32. Thomas EJ, Campbell IG. Molecular genetic defects in endometriosis. Gynecol Obstet Invest 2000;50(suppl 1):44–50
33. Van Gorp T, Amant F, Neven P et al. Endometriosis and the development of malignant tumours of the pelvis. A review of literature. Best Pract Res Clin Obstet Gynaecol 2004;18:349–371
34. Cornillie FJ, Oosterlynck D, Lauweryns JM, Koninckx PR. Deeply infiltrating pelvic endometriosis: histology and clinical significance. Fertil Steril 1990;53:978–983
35. Koninckx PR, Meuleman C, Demeyere S et al. Suggestive evidence that pelvic endometriosis is a progressive disease, whereas deeply infiltrating endometriosis is associated with pelvic pain. Fertil Steril 1991;55:759–765
36. Vercellini P, Frontino G, Pietropaolo G et al. Deep endometriosis: definition, pathogenesis,

and clinical management. J Am Assoc Gynecol Laparosc 2004;11:153–161
37. Koninckx PR, Oosterlynck D, D'Hooghe T, Meuleman C. Deeply infiltrating endometriosis is a disease whereas mild endometriosis could be considered a non-disease. Ann N Y Acad Sci 1994;734:333–341
38. Nisolle M, Donnez J. Peritoneal endometriosis, ovarian endometriosis, and adenomyotic nodules of the rectovaginal septum are three different entities. Fertil Steril 1997;68:585–596
39. Koninckx PR, Martin DC. Deep endometriosis: a consequence of infiltration or retraction or possibly adenomyosis externa? Fertil Steril 1992;58:924–928
40. Nakamura M, Katabuchi H, Tohya TR et al. Scanning electron microscopic and immunohistochemical studies of pelvic endometriosis. Hum Reprod 1993;8:2218–2226
41. Donnez J, Nisolle M. L'endométriose péritonéale, le kyste endométriotique ovarien et le nodule de la lame rectovaginale sont trois pathologies différentes [editorial]. Ref Gynecol Obstet 1995;3:121–123
42. Donnez J, Nisolle M, Smoes P et al. Peritoneal endometriosis and "endometriotic" nodules of the rectovaginal septum are two different entities. Fertil Steril 1996;66:362–368
43. Vercellini P, Aimi G, De Giorgi O et al. Is cystic ovarian endometriosis an asymmetric disease? Br J Obstet Gynaecol 1998;105:1018–1021
44. Vercellini P, Busacca M, Aimi G et al. Lateral distribution of recurrent ovarian endometriotic cysts. Fertil Steril 2002;77:848–849
45. Vercellini P, Frontino G, Pisacreta A et al. The pathogenesis of bladder detrusor endometriosis. Am J Obstet Gynecol 2002;187:538–542
46. Somigliana E, Infantino M, Candiani M et al. Association rate between deep peritoneal endometriosis and other forms of the disease: pathogenetic implications. Hum Reprod 2004;19:168–171
47. Somigliana E, Vercellini P, Gattei U et al. Bladder endometriosis: getting closer and closer to the unifying metastatic hypothesis. Fertil Steril 2007;87:1287–1290
48. Bricou A, Batt RE, Chapron C. Peritoneal fluid flow influences anatomical distribution of endometriotic lesions: why Sampson seems to be right. Eur J Obstet Gynecol Reprod Biol 2008;138:127–134
49. Chapron C, Chopin N, Borghese B et al. Deeply infiltrating endometriosis: pathogenetic implications of the anatomical distribution. Hum Reprod 2006;21:1839–1845
50. Brosens IA, Puttemans P, Deprest J, Rombauts L. The endometriosis cycle and its derailments. Hum Reprod 1994;9:770–771
51. Vercellini P, Meschia M, De Giorgi O et al. Bladder detrusor endometriosis: clinical and pathogenetic implications. J Urol 1996;155:84–86
52. Al-Fozan H, Tulandi T. Left lateral predisposition of endometriosis and endometrioma. Obstet Gynecol 2003;101:164–166
53. Parazzini F. Left: right side ratio of endometriotic implants in the pelvis. Eur J Obstet Gynecol Reprod Biol 2003;111:65–67
54. Sznurkowski J, Emerich J. Left lateral predisposition of endometrioma. Ginekol Pol 2005,76:33–36
55. Meyers MA. Distribution of intra-abdominal malignant seeding: dependency on dynamics of flow of ascitic fluid. Am J Roentgenol Radium Ther Nucl Med 1973;119:198–206
56. Martin DC, Batt RE. Retrocervical, retrovaginal pouch, and rectovaginal septum endometriosis. J Am Assoc Gynecol Laparosc 2001;8:12–17
57. Bonte H, Chapron C, Vieira M et al. Histologic appearance of endometriosis infiltrating uterosacral ligaments in women with painful symptoms. J Am Assoc Gynecol Laparosc 2002;9:519–524
58. Chapron C, Liaras E, Fayet P et al. Magnetic resonance imaging and endometriosis: deeply infiltrating endometriosis does not originate from the rectovaginal septum. Gynecol Obstet Invest 2002;53:204–208

59. De Lancey JOL. Surgical anatomy of the female pelvis. In: Rock JA, Thompson JD (eds) The Linde's operative gynecology, 8 edn. Lippincott-Raven, Philadelphia (PA), 1997, pp 63–93
60. Kuhn RJ, Hollyock VE. Observations on the anatomy of the rectovaginal pouch and septum. Obstet Gynecol 1982;59:445–447
61. Baessler K, Schuessler B. The depth of the pouch of Douglas in nulliparous and parous women without genital prolapse and in patients with genital prolapse. Am J Obstet Gynecol 2000;182:540–544
62. Anaf V, Simon P, Fayt I, Noel J. Smooth muscles are frequent components of endometriotic lesions. Hum Reprod 2000;15:767–771
63. Classification of endometriosis. The American Fertility Society. Fertil Steril 1979;32:633–634
64. Revised American Fertility Society Classification of endometriosis: 1985. Fertil Steril 1985;43:351–352
65. Vercellini P, Vendola N, Bocciolone L et al. Reliability of the visual diagnosis of ovarian endometriosis. Fertil Steril 1991;56:1198–1200
66. Martin DC (ed). Laparoscopic appearance of endometriosis, 2 edn. Resurge Press, Memphis (TN), 1991
67. Jenkins S, Olive DL, Haney AF. Endometriosis: pathogenetic implications of the anatomic distribution. Obstet Gynecol 1986;67:335–338
68. Adamyan LV. Additional international perspectives. In: Nichols DH (ed) Gynecologic and obstetric surgery. Mosby, St Louis (MO), 1993, pp 1167–1182
69. Chapron C, Fauconnier A, Vieira M et al. Anatomical distribution of deeply infiltrating endometriosis: surgical implications and proposition for a classification. Hum Reprod 2003;18:157–161

Diagnosis

2

P. De Nardi, S. Ferrari

Abstract Symptoms of endometriosis are extremely nonspecific and variable, with considerable overlap with other conditions, and difficult to interpret, thus causing delay in diagnosis. Pain is the most common symptom that may be associated with urinary or gastrointestinal complaints. Physical findings are variable and depend on the location and size of the implants.

Traditionally, laparoscopy has been the preferred method to diagnose endometriosis; however, in the presence of adhesion, the real extension of the disease into the subperitoneal space may not be adequately predicted. Imaging methods are therefore mandatory, with the aim of diagnosing every possible implant, planning the surgical procedure, and informing the patient about the possible results and complications of surgical resection.

To date, no definitive guidelines exist for the preoperative assessment of deep pelvic endometriosis. Abdominal and transvaginal ultrasonography are the initial investigations and may be adequate when medical treatment is recommended. When a more precise definition of the extent of the disease is needed, with a view to surgical treatment, other imaging modalities are employed. Endorectal ultrasound is useful when bowel wall infiltration is suspected. Computerized tomography

P. De Nardi (✉)
Department of Surgery, San Raffaele Scientific Institute, Milan, Italy

Deep Pelvic Endometriosis. Paola De Nardi, Stefano Ferrari

allows a complete staging of all pelvic endometriotic lesions but has been substituted by magnetic resonance imaging because of the high accuracy and noninvasiveness of this alternative. Finally, cystoscopy, intravenous pyelography, and ureteroscopy are recommended for all patients with endometriosis and lower urinary tract symptoms.

Keywords Pain • Dysmenorrhea • Ultrasonography • MRI

2.1 Clinical Features

Endometriosis is a common gynecologic disease. Women affected by endometriosis claim that the delay in diagnosis is a great problem. This problem has been discussed since 1996 when Hadfiel et al reported an average delay of 11.7 years in the USA and 8.0 years in the UK from the onset of pain symptoms until the time of diagnosis [1]. The median delay from pain debut to diagnosis for both groups was 7.5 years. This delay in diagnosis is still a widespread problem and causes a long period of pain, uncertainty, and distrust. Moreover, an early diagnosis means that specific treatment can be initiated. In addition, the patient can be made aware of her subfertility and can choose from a selection of contraceptive methods for family planning that may reduce the activity and growth of endometriosis.

This problem in establishing the diagnosis of endometriosis is due to difficulties in interpreting the presenting symptoms. The presentation is highly variable, the symptoms are extremely nonspecific, and there is considerable overlap with other conditions, such as irritable bowel syndrome and pelvic inflammatory disease.

2.2 Symptoms

Pain is the most common symptom associated with endometriosis. Approximately three-quarters of symptomatic patients experience pelvic pain and/or dysmenorrhea [2]. The following symptoms can be caused by endometriosis, based on clinical and patient experience [2, 3]:

- severe dysmenorrhea;
- pelvic pain;
- deep dyspareunia;
- cyclical or perimenstrual gastrointestinal or urologic symptoms;
- pain at defecation or micturition;
- subfertility;
- abnormal menstrual bleeding;
- chronic fatigue;
- backache.

These symptoms are also present in other disorders such as pelvic inflammatory disease, irritable bowel syndrome, interstitial cystitis, adenomyosis, ovarian neoplasms, pelvic adhesions, colon cancer, and diverticular disease [4], as well as in unaffected women. This causes even more difficulties concerning differential diagnosis and rapid selection of endometriotic patients. For example, a national case-control study found that 73% of women with endometriosis reported abdominopelvic pain, dysmenorrhea, or menorrhagia, but 20% of matched controls without endometriosis also reported these symptoms [5]. On the other hand, many women with endometriosis are completely asymptomatic.

It is known that the extent of the disease varies from few, small lesions on otherwise normal pelvic organs, to large, ovarian endometriotic cysts (endometriomas) and/or extensive fibrosis and adhesion formation causing marked distortion of pelvic anatomy. It has been demonstrated that there is no correlation between the extent of the disease and type or severity of pain symptoms [6–8]. As commonly observed by patients, pelvic pain may be chronic, but is often more severe during menses or at ovulation, and furthermore it may be more common and severe in women with deep infiltrating endometriosis (DIE) implants [9, 10]. In particular, severe deep dyspareunia and painful defecation during menses are suggestive of posterior deep infiltrating disease [11].

The relationship between pelvic pain and endometriosis appears to be very complex. To illustrate this, animal experiments have suggested that the location and innervation patterns of the endometrial deposits are probably more important for nociception than the visual extent of disease [12].

A recent study has demonstrated that a range of nerve fibers are found at high density in peritoneal endometriotic lesions, including sensory C, sensory Aδ, cholinergic, and adrenergic nerve fibers [13, 14]. Although the mechanisms stimulating increased nerve fiber density in endometriotic lesions are still unclear, it is likely that these nerves have a crucial role in the generation of pain in endometriosis.

The relationship between subfertility and disease stage is similarly uncertain. In fact, the mechanism for subfertility may involve anatomic distortion from pelvic adhesions and endometriomas and/or production of substances (for example, prostanoids, cytokines, and growth factors) that are "hostile" to normal ovarian function/ovulation, fertilization, and implantation [15].

Urinary tract involvement in patients with endometriosis is relatively uncommon and occurs in approximately 1–2% of cases; the bladder is the most frequently involved organ, followed by the ureters and kidneys, in a ratio of 40:5:1 [16]. Ureteral endometriosis can be classified as extrinsic or intrinsic. Intrinsic ureteral endometriosis, characterized by the presence of endometriotic glands and stroma in the ureteral wall, is rare. Extrinsic ureteral endometriosis, which is caused by extraureteral disease, is more frequent.

Donnez et al reported a prevalence of 88% of their patients presenting with pure extrinsic ureteral endometriosis. Surrounding endometriotic lesions responsible for external ureteral compression, without histological evidence of endometriotic glands and stroma in the ureteral wall, are thus mostly due to lateral extension of rectovaginal endometriotic (adenomyotic) nodules. About 11% of patients presented both extrinsic and intrinsic ureteral endometriosis. Histological analysis of the removed ureteral segment revealed glands in the ureteral wall up to the lumen [16]. It cannot be excluded that the two forms constitute different degrees of the same histopathogenetic process.

Similarly to ovarian endometriosis, ureteral disease is observed more frequently on the left than the right side. Interestingly, the proportions of left-sided gonad and ureteral lesions are remarkably similar (63–64%) [17]. However, endometriosis of the ureters may not necessarily be secondary to endometriotic cysts only, but more generally to ectopic implantation of endometrial cells along the lateral gonad aspect and ovarian fossa. Indeed, the asymmetry of both ovarian and ureteral forms may be the expression of a common underlying anatomical condition that facilitates adhesion and growth of endometrial cells on the left pelvic side wall [17].

Patients with ureteral endometriosis often refer to nonspecific symptoms at clinical presentation, therefore posing differential diagnostic problems and a relatively high risk for subsequent loss of renal function. In a small number of these patients, the presence of a renal colic will lead to prompt diagnosis and thus to an earlier treatment. Carmignani et al reported that the high rate of asymptomatic ureteral involvement (56.5%) in patients with known pelvic endometriosis seems to warrant the need for further investigations regarding the possibility of avoiding the high percentage of silent renal losses [17]. The loss of renal units in patients with ureteral endometriosis causing hydronephrosis has been estimated to be 25–50% at the time of diagnosis, although these data derive from limited case series.

Patients with suspected or proven pelvic endometriosis should systematically undergo a sonographic kidney evaluation during routine gynecological sonographic examination. It remains to be evaluated whether urinary ultrasound ensures a beneficial cost/benefit ratio if used on a routine basis, especially concerning the relatively large patient numbers.

Obstructive uropathy should be suspected in patients with a rectovaginal endometriotic nodule larger than 3 cm, because of its high prevalence. Intravenous pyelography should be performed in those considered at risk for obstructive uropathy before the laparoscopic procedure is done, including ureterolysis and removal of associated DIE lesions [16].

2.3 Physical Findings

Physical findings in women with endometriosis are variable and depend upon the location and size of the implants [18]. There are often no abnormal findings on physical examination. When findings are present, lesions may be visualized on the posterior vaginal fornix; infiltration or a nodule is detected on vaginal examination, involving the vagina, torus uterinus, uterosacral ligaments, or pouch of Douglas, and infiltration or a mass is detected on rectal digital examination. Thickening and induration of the uterosacral ligaments may be also present, possibly even as a single element of suspicion. Pain may be evoked by movement of the uterus, or fixation of the uterus in a retroverted position may be detected [19]. The accuracy of physical examination is usually higher if performed during menstruation; however, it has limited value in the prediction of extension of the disease. Bazot correlated the result of physical examination to other noninvasive diagnostic techniques: physical examination correctly diagnosed deep pelvic infiltration (DIE) in 81.5% of women, but specific involvement of the uterosacral ligaments, rectosigmoid, rectum, or rectovaginal septum was diagnosed in a low proportion of cases (68.5%, 40.2%, 25%) [20].

2.4 Serum Markers

Endometrial cells express the antigen CA 125, an epitope that has been demonstrated to be associated with coelomic epithelium and its neoplastic derivatives. Since Barbieri et al [21] demonstrated elevated serum concentrations of CA 125 in patients with advanced endometriosis, various investigators have suggested that this antigen can be used as a marker for endometriosis [22, 23].

However, the results of studies comparing CA 125 and CA 19.9 levels in patients with endometriosis are still contradictory [24–26]. One study has reported significantly higher levels of CA 19.9 antigen and its correlation to severity of the disease [21]. The other studies revealed that patients with endometriosis had significantly higher levels of CA 125, but they failed to show that CA 19.9 can be used to discriminate between patients with or without endometriosis, even in combination with CA 125 [22, 23]. Harada et al [24] found that the sensitivity of the CA 19.9 test (34%) was statistically significantly lower than that of the CA 125 test (49%), whereas there was no difference in the positive and negative likelihood ratios between these two tests in the diagnosis of endometriosis. In a more recent study, Kurdoglu et al [27] observed a positive correlation between serum CA 125 and CA 19.9 levels with revised American Fertility Association (r-AFS) scores. They observed that patients with stage III endometriosis had significantly higher levels of CA 125 and CA 19.9 as compared to patients without endometriosis. However, serum CA 125 and CA 19.9 levels were not different in patients with stage I and II endometriosis as compared to patients without endometriosis. Serum CA 125 and CA 19.9 levels were also significantly higher in patients with stage III and IV endometriosis as compared to patients with stage I endometriosis. These findings suggest that endometriosis may be the source of high CA 19.9 levels. In fact, immunostaining properties of the cases reported by Kurdoglu et al [27] verify that endometriotic tissues were the origin of these tumor markers. In conclusion, the data of the current studies reveal that both CA 125 and CA 19.9 have high sensitivity with relatively low specificity in the detection of endometriosis. However, the predictive values of CA 125 and CA 19.9 seem only to be high for severe (stages III and IV) disease.

2.5 Laparoscopy

Laparoscopy is considered the gold standard for diagnosis and evaluation of the extent of abdominal endometriosis; in fact, during laparoscopy the presence and size of ovarian endometrioma, peritoneal implants, and tubal adhesion can be correctly staged. However, exploratory laparoscopy where the cul-de-sac cannot always be explored, can barely diagnose rectovaginal endometriosis. In the presence of adhesion, operative laparoscopy, with opening of the subperitoneal space, may be required. Even so, the real extent of the disease, especially rectal wall infiltration, may not be accurately predicted [28].

2.6 Instrumental Diagnosis

Since an accurate mapping of DIE, including the extent of intestinal and urologic involvement, is essential for surgical treatment, imaging methods are mandatory to improve the noninvasive diagnosis. The presence of intestinal and urological involvement should be investigated in all patients with pelvic endometriosis, and in those with rectovaginal septum lesions it is necessary to exclude possible infiltration of the rectal wall [29].

If it is determined before surgery whether the bowel muscular layer is infiltrated by endometriosis, the gynecologist can discuss the surgical approach (nodulectomy or bowel resection) with the colorectal surgeon. Furthermore, determining the presence and extent of rectal nodules allows informed consent to be obtained from the patient; this consent is particularly relevant when rectal resection is required, because the risk of complications increases.

Many techniques have been suggested to be useful for preoperative diagnosis of DIE, and all of them are still used although no single one is yet considered as a gold standard.

The goals of the imaging technique are to:

- diagnose all possible implants;
- aid in planning the surgical procedure;
- inform the patient about the possible results and complications of surgical resection.

As seen before, in patients with endometriosis of the posterior cul-de-sac, endometriotic implants may cause painful narrowing of the rectosigmoid lumen and ureteral obstruction. Rectal blood loss occurs only rarely [30]. Narrowing of the colonic lumen may eventually lead to complete large-bowel obstruction, whereas ureteral obstruction may lead to complete loss of renal function.

Physical examination may show a firm pelvic mass, but this finding is not sufficient for the diagnosis of posterior cul-de-sac endometriosis [31].

2.6.1 Abdominal Ultrasonography

Abdominal ultrasonography (US) is the initial investigation of choice in evaluation of dysmenorrhea or a pelvic mass, because of its low cost, ready availability, and lack of radiation exposure [32]. It may reveal coexisting endometrial cysts and hydronephrosis, but it rarely detects relatively small and deeply located endometrial implants in the pouch of Douglas. In the case of bladder endometriosis, US has proved to be adequate in determining the site and size of lesion, the degree of infiltration of the detrusor and mucosa, the cleavage plane between the detrusor lesion and the uterine wall, and, consequently, the relationship with concomitant adenomyosis of the uterus [33, 34]. In addition, US has shown good specificity (88%) in evaluating the uterosacral ligaments and posterior compartment for endometriotic lesions. Despite these indications, its low sensitivity (64%) limits the usefulness of US for early diagnosis [35].

US is routinely used as a screening tool to rule out urinary tract obstruction in patients with pelvic endometriosis. In fact, patients with suspected or proven pelvic endometriosis should systematically undergo a sonographic kidney evaluation during routine gynecological US examination, due to the high rate of silent presentations [36]. Moreover, early diagnosis of hydronephrosis is critical to preserve renal function in these young patients, rather than considering eventual therapeutic strategies.

2.6.2 Transvaginal Sonography

Transvaginal sonography (TVS) is the most common examination; since it is often available at the time of gynecological consultation it should be considered the most accessible imaging method. The examination is carried out and interpreted in real time and is relatively inexpensive. It has few disadvantages, among which are that it cannot be performed on virgins or patients with genital malformations. The characteristics of DIE at transvaginal ultrasound have been described as a heterogeneous, hypo-echoic, sometimes speculated mass arising from the serosal surface of the rectosigmoid [37, 38] (Fig. 2.1). It appears as a solid and noncompressible mass, and shows minimal internal vascularity on power Doppler imaging, reflecting the fibrotic character of the lesion.

TVS has been extensively employed for the diagnosis of endometrioma but less frequently in DIE, in particular for posterior involvement. Nevertheless, in expert hands it may correctly diagnose rectosigmoid and uterosacral involvement in a high percentage of cases. A prospective study by Bazot et al [29] suggested that TVS can demonstrate the infiltration of the muscularis propria, which is normally hypo-echoic and thin (<3 mm), replaced by the abnormal tissue mass. This study showed a sensitivity of TVS of about 95.5%, with 100% specificity, a positive predictive value (PPV) of 100%, and a negative predictive value (NPV) of 88.9%.

In a more recent study, the same authors demonstrated that TVS presents a higher accuracy than transrectal echoendoscopy in the diagnosis of rectal endometriosis [39]. The efficacy of TVS has also been confirmed by other authors [19].

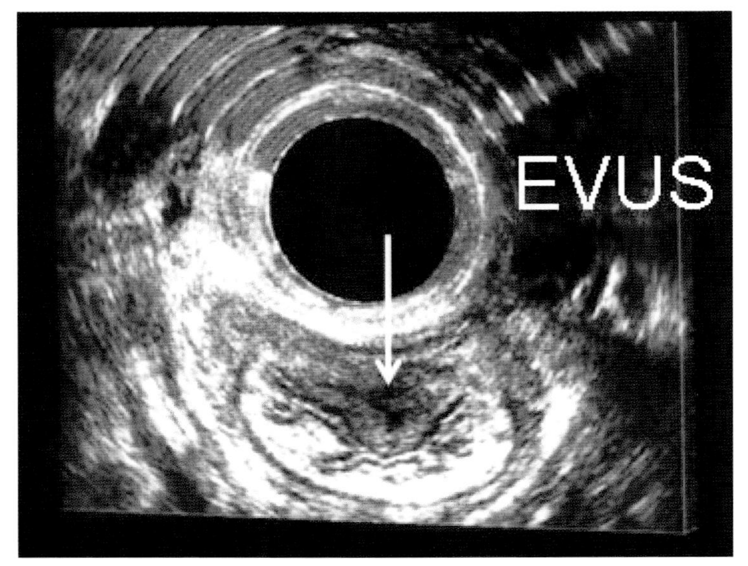

Fig. 2.1 Transvaginal ultrasound image: endometriotic nodule in the rectovaginal space (*arrow*), invading the rectal wall from the outside (provided courtesy of Dr Santoro)

The information obtained by TVS has definite limitations, and additional imaging such as abdominal ultrasonography, barium enema, rectosigmoidoscopy, computerized tomography (CT), or magnetic resonance imaging (MRI) is needed, especially in the assessment of posterior cul-de-sac endometriosis. However, TVS is simple, cheap, fast, and less invasive than some other examinations [31, 38].

2.6.3 Rectal Water-contrast Transvaginal Sonography

It has recently been suggested that rectal distension with water-contrast during TVS may help to determine the depth of infiltration of the nodules that locate in the rectovaginal septum, and can easily distinguish between the involved bowel layers because of its high spatial resolution in the near field, which is an advantage over other imaging techniques. The sensitivity of this technique for detecting rectal lesions reaching the muscular layer has been shown to be 100%, with 85.7% specificity, a PPV of 91.3%, and NPV of 100% [40]. The results shown by Valenzano Menada et al [40] indicate that adding water-contrast to the rectum improves the identification of rectal infiltration reaching at least as far as the muscular layer. Rectal water-contrast transvaginal sonography (RWC-TVS) identified 22 out of 23 cases of rectal infiltration (sensitivity 95.7%); infiltration of the rectal muscular layer is particularly relevant because it may increase the risks of postoperative complications if the endometriotic nodule is completely excised [40].

The use of RWC-TVS in diagnosing rectal infiltration in women with rectovaginal endometriosis has several potential advantages over other techniques. First, TVS is a simple technique that has high diffusion, and it is usually performed by gynecologists; the longitudinal images obtained at RWC-TVS are more familiar to the gynecologist than those obtained by rectal endoscopic ultrasonography (EUS). Secondly, this examination can be easily performed in any gynecological department, while the equipment for EUS is often unavailable. Thirdly, RWC-TVS is less invasive than other examinations (such as rectal EUS) that sometimes necessitate general anesthesia. Fourthly, RWC-TVS may provide information on the distensibility of the intestinal walls: this information could be useful for the surgeon because distensibility may reflect endometriosis-associated fibrosis present in the intestinal wall.

A limitation of RWC-TVS is that it is unsuitable for diagnosing endometriotic nodules located above the rectosigmoid junction, which are beyond the field of view of ultrasonography. Furthermore, the bowel distension may be uncomfortable for patients and should be used only in those patients with uncertain intestinal involvement.

2.6.4 Sonovaginography

Another water-contrast variant of TVS is sonovaginography, which consists of transvaginal ultrasonography combined with the introduction of saline solution to the vagina. In this way, an acoustic window is formed between the transvaginal probe and the surrounding structures of the vaginal channel, that is, the vaginal fornix, the vaginal walls, rectovaginal septum, uterosacral ligaments, and vescicovaginal septum.

With this technique, endometriotic lesions are detected as hypo-echoic, irregular structures at the level of the vaginal wall; they often infiltrate the surrounding structures and the uterosacral ligaments. On the basis of the images collected using this method, Dessole et al [41] classified the endometriotic lesions as follows: esophitic, infiltrating, plaque, and mixed lesions. Esophitic lesions were defined as structures originating from the vaginal wall and protruding into the vaginal channel; infiltrating lesions were structures extending through the vaginal wall, reaching the vescico-vaginal or rectovaginal septum and/or pouch of Douglas; plaque lesions were defined as structures confined to within the vaginal wall; and mixed lesions were those that presented more than one of the above lesions' characteristics.

The results of sonovaginography, compared with surgical and pathologic findings, enabled the detection of rectovaginal endometriosis with high sensitivity (90.6%); moreover, the method showed excellent sensitivity in evaluating the location and extent of the different types of endometriotic lesions in the vaginal wall (100%). Furthermore, patient compliance was similar in both techniques.

Even with this technique, however, the greatest limitation of TVS is the impossibility of investigating lesions that are proximal to the rectosigmoid junction [41].

2.6.5 "Tenderness-guided" Ultrasonography

As an alternative, in 2007 Guerriero et al [42] created a new modality of ultrasonographic evaluation called "tenderness-guided" ultrasonography; using an acoustic window between the transvaginal probe and the surrounding vaginal structures by increasing the amount of ultrasound gel inside the probe cover, coupled with an "active" role of the patient, who indicated the site of any tenderness experienced during examination, this method seems to improve the diagnostic accuracy. The use of this efficient but noninvasive technique with no associated discomfort, may not only decrease the waiting time for a laparoscopy, but also, in some cases, avoid laparoscopy if it is too risky, as in the case of a rectosigmoid involvement, and hence permit an effective medical therapy based on the administration of low-cost drugs such as oral contraceptives [43].

2.6.6 Three-dimensional Transvaginal Ultrasonography

A few studies have evaluated the potential role of three-dimensional ultrasonography (3DUS) in the preoperative work-up of DIE. Seow et al [44] reported that transvaginal 3DUS was suitable for evaluating the adhesions in women with surgically proven pelvic adhesions. They also found that sensitivity increased when sonographic findings were combined with abnormalities in the serum level of CA 125.

In a very recent study, Grasso et al [45] showed that the surface-rendering mode allows recognition of benign lesion features showing the surface "regularity" of endometriomas. Transparent maximum/minimum mode can be adopted in differential diagnosis with tumors or dermoid cysts because of a better visualization of intratumoral calcifications and bone abnormalities (typical of dermoid cysts). Power and color Doppler support the diagnosis of endometriomas in showing a typical vascular location: regularly separated pericystic vessels with low or moderate vascular resistance.

The uterosacral ligaments can be considered involved when they appear thickened in 3D scans, or show a regular or irregular hypo-echogenic nodule near their insertion on the cervix. Posterior vaginal fornix involvement can be seen as a cystic or thickened area. Such abnormalities can also be seen in the rectovaginal septum under the horizontal plane passing through the posterior lip of the cervix, under the peritoneum. Sigmoid colon involvement is diagnosed when a hypo-echoic area with irregular margins penetrates into bowel walls. Deep bladder endometriosis can appear as iso-echogenic or hypo-echogenic nodules or cystic lesions in the bladder wall, and can be differentiated from endometriosis foci in the uterovescical fold.

In the study by Grasso et al [45], the sensitivity and specificity of 3DUS for uterosacral involvement were 50% and 94.7% respectively, while for posterior vaginal fornix infiltration they were 84% and 80% respectively.

Rectovaginal septum endometriosis and sigmoid colon endometriosis were diagnosed with a sensitivity of 76.9% and 33.3% respectively, and the specificity was 100% in both cases. For bladder endometriosis, the sensitivity was 25% and specificity 100%.

TVS is the first-line imaging method in patients with pelvic disorders and shows high degrees of accuracy in the diagnosis of endometrial lesions. 3DUS can help the investigator in evaluation of lesions by a scrupulous morphologic analysis; it also reduces the number of false-positive diagnoses when analyzing complex lesions such as endometrial cysts, ovarian dermoids, fibromas, and corpus luteum cysts, which may give a wrong impression of malignancy when using conventional TVS [45].

2.6.7 Endoscopic Transrectal Ultrasonography

Endoscopic transrectal ultrasonography (EUS) has been introduced for studying rectal cancer and inflammatory perineal disease. Recently it has also been applied to the diagnostic approach of DIE. EUS can be performed by two methods. The first one is transrectal ultrasound with a rigid, 360° circulating probe; this examination is usually performed by the surgeon during coloproctological consultation (Figs. 2. 2 and 2.3). The second method is the use of an echoendoscope, that is, an endoscope equipped with a transducer on its tip; this instrument is flexible and generally has a lower diameter, thus

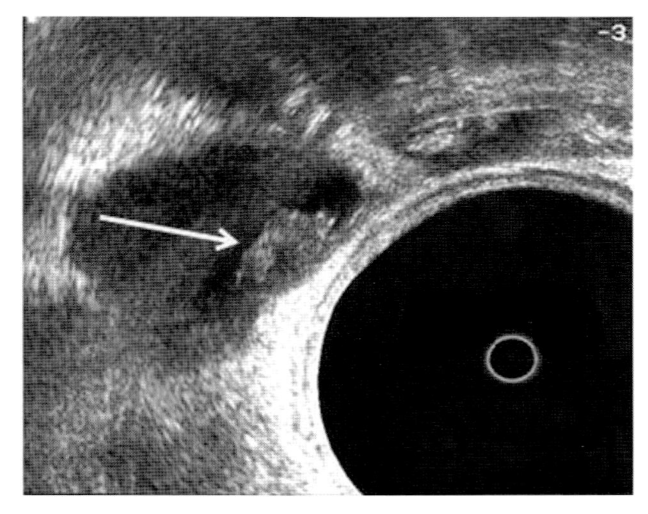

Fig. 2.2 Endorectal ultrasonography with a rotating probe. Endometriotic nodule invading the muscularis layer of the intraperitoneal rectum (*arrow*) (provided courtesy of Dr Santoro)

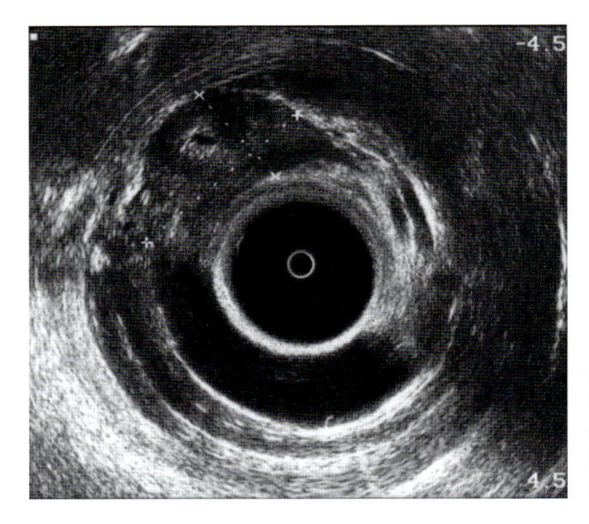

Fig. 2.3 Endorectal ultrasonography with a rotating probe. Endometriotic nodule of the rectovaginal space invading the muscularis and submucosal layer of the rectal wall

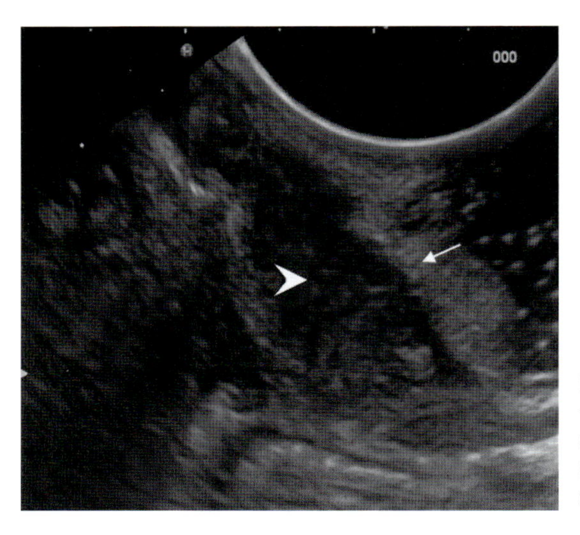

Fig. 2.4 Endoscopic ultrasonography with echoendoscope: hypo-echoic endometriosis (*arrowhead*) invading the muscularis of the rectal wall, reaching the submucosa (*arrow*)

allowing inclusion of a substenotic area, and reaching the sigmoid colon, an area that is frequently involved in intestinal endometriosis (Fig. 2.4). The majority of published studies have employed this instrument. The echoendoscope is usually advanced up to the sigmoid colon and then withdrawn while studying the bowel wall; the entire examination lasts approximately 15–20 min. This examination can be executed without anesthesia with a previous intestinal preparation by small enema, although some authors prefer general anesthesia [29].

EUS transducers, using higher frequencies than TVS transducers, allow good definition of the bowel-wall layers but a narrow view (limited to a few centimeters) of adjacent pelvic organs. Chapron et al [46] showed that EUS permits the diagnosis of intestinal endometriosis with a sensitivity of 97.1%, specificity 89.4%, PPV 86.8%, and NPV 97.7%. At EUS, DIE is visible as a hypo-echoic nodule or mass, with or without regular contours.

The principal advantage is that the EUS can accurately predict the involvement of each of the five layers of the bowel wall, in particular the infiltration of the muscularis propria. In just one study, the depth of rectal wall infiltration was overestimated in 30% of cases, but in the majority of studies EUS has been considered reliable and recommended. Another important piece of information given by EUS is the exact distance between the rectal lesion and the anal margin. This information is essential for planning the surgical resection and to predict possible complications and sequelae. Moreover, in patients with rectal involvement we have observed a correlation between several echoendoscopic findings, such as a nodule greater than 3 cm, or more than two nodules invading the rectal wall, and the need for surgical treatment.

Although highly accurate in the diagnosis of intestinal endometriosis, with an elevated sensitivity and specificity in definition of the compromised intestinal layer, EUS has some limitations. Its use is still restricted to some centers; the equipment and expertise for this test are not yet widely available; the costs are high and, as for other ultrasonographic tests, its reproducibility is low. One of the main drawbacks is the unbearable pain elicited by the examination, which is described by some patients, with a consequent need for sedation or general anesthesia. However, in our experience, no general anesthesia is required and all patients complete the examination without problems, with a light sedation. Furthermore, EUS can accurately diagnose posterior pelvic lesions, although it may miss anterior pelvic lesions and has poor sensitivity for the diagnosis of endometriomas and obliteration of the pouch of Douglas. Very recently, ultrasound elastography has gained considerable interest as a method to separate normal from pathological tissue. Its usefulness in determining the microscopic infiltration of the bowel wall is currently being evaluated (Fig. 2.5).

In our experience, as the overall accuracy of TVS and EUS is similar, EUS seems to be indicated when colorectal involvement is strongly suspected.

In an interesting study by Bazot et al [29], a strong relationship was found between histology and TVS, in relation to the maximum diameter of colorectal lesions. In contrast, EUS often underestimated the overall size of colorectal lesions. This discrepancy could be explained by the low accuracy

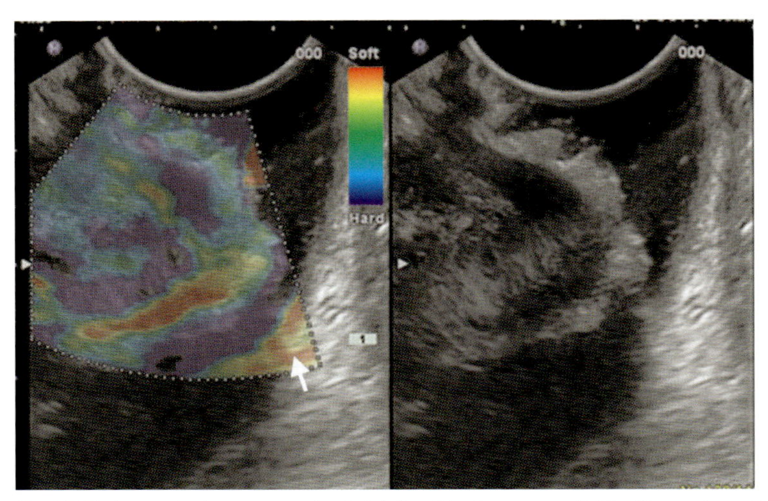

Fig. 2.5 Endorectal ultrasonography (**right**) with elastogram (**left**). The endometriotic nodule is blue while the mucosa and submucosal layer are colored in yellow and red (*arrow*)

of EUS for assessing the lateral extent of endometriosis, especially that involving the uterosacral ligaments, which are often fibrotic in this setting. From the clinical point of view, the data of Bazot et al underline that TVS and EUS have similar accuracy for the diagnosis of colorectal endometriosis. From the surgical point of view, their data confirm that one advantage of EUS is its ability to determine the distance of colorectal lesions from the anal margins when segmental resection is required.

Therefore, when medical treatment option is recommended, TVS examination may be sufficient. However, in our opinion, when surgical treatment is planned, this opportunity to use EUS should not be missed, in order to correctly inform the patient about the risks of bowel, and particularly rectal, resection.

2.6.8 Magnetic Resonance Imaging

Magnetic Resonance Imaging (MRI) has also been used for the diagnosis of DIE. The role of MRI for the evaluation of pelvic endometriosis was firstly reported by Siegelman et al [46]. In a recent study, MRI demonstrated high sensitivity, specificity, PPV, NPV, and accuracy in the prediction of locations and extension of the disease in patients with deep pelvic endometriosis (sensitivity 90.3%; specificity 91%; PPV 92.1%; NPV 89%) [45]. The diagnosis of DIE with MRI is based on the combined presence of morphologic abnormalities and signal abnormalities, such as hyperintense foci on T_1-weighted or fat-suppression T_1-weighted MRIs (Figs 2.6 and 2.7), corresponding to hemorrhagic foci or small hyperintense cavities on T_2-weighted images, or areas corresponding to fibrosis, with a signal close to that of pelvic muscle on T_1- and T_2-weighted images, with or without foci or cavities, and with or without contrast enhancement after gadolinium injection [47].

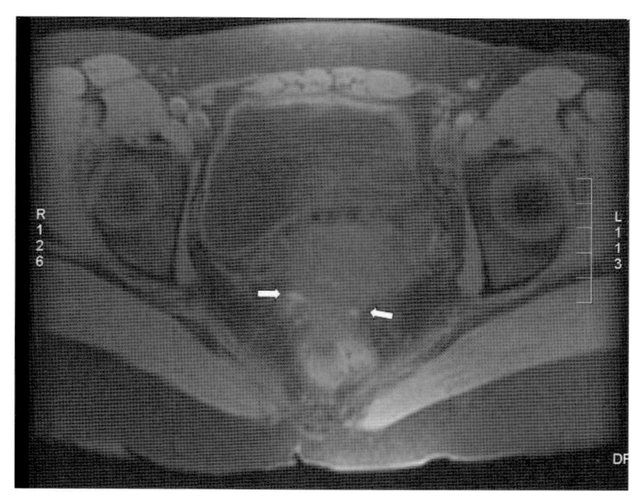

Fig. 2.6 MRI, fat-suppression T_1-weighted imaging of two hyperintense foci (*arrows*) of small endometriotic hemorrhagic nodules of the rectovaginal septum

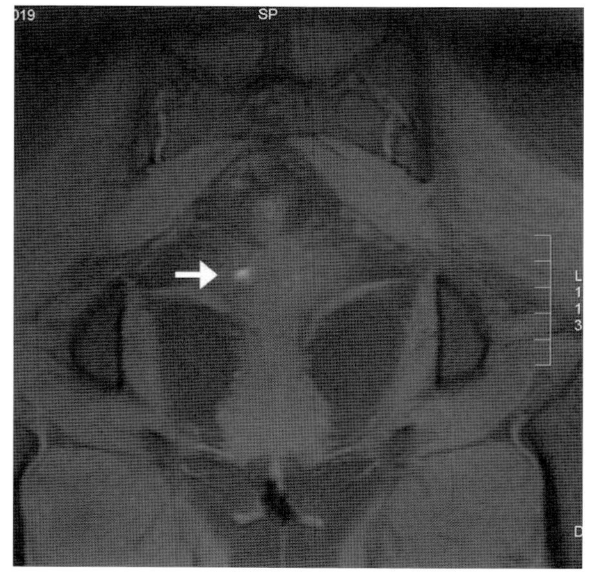

Fig. 2.7 Same case as Fig. 2.6, MRI, fat-suppression T_1-weighted imaging, coronal plane

Uterosacral ligament endometriosis is visible as a nodule (regular or stellate margins) or a fibrotic thickening compared with the contralateral uterosacral ligament, with regular or irregular margins. The unilateral/bilateral nature of the involvement of the torus uterinus (aciform abnormality) can be observed. Vaginal endometriosis is defined by obliteration of the hypointense signal of the posterior vaginal wall on T_2-weighted images, with thickening or a mass (containing or not containing foci) behind the posterior wall of the cervix.

Rectovaginal septum lesion is defined by a nodule or a mass passing through the lower border of the posterior lip of the cervix (under the peritoneum). Rectosigmoid colon endometriosis is defined by disappearance of the fat tissue plane lying between the uterus and the rectum/sigmoid colon, and its replacement by a tissue mass, and by disappearance of the hypointense signal of the anterior wall of the rectum/sigmoid colon on T_2-weighted images, with contrast enhancement on T_1-weighted images (Figs. 2.8 and 2.9).

Localized bladder wall thickening occasionally protruding inside the bladder lumen represents the main diagnostic criterion of anterior-compartment endometriosis. It appears iso-intense on T_2-weighted images and with hyperintense spots on T_1-weighted sequences (Fig. 2.10).

Ureteral endometriosis is detectable on T_2-weighted sequences as a hypointense nodule associated with hyperintense foci close to the ureter on both T_1- and T_2-weighted images. Our imaging protocol includes: T_2-weighted sequences in different slice orientations; T_1-weighted sequences in an identical imaging plane that best demonstrates the endometriotic localization,

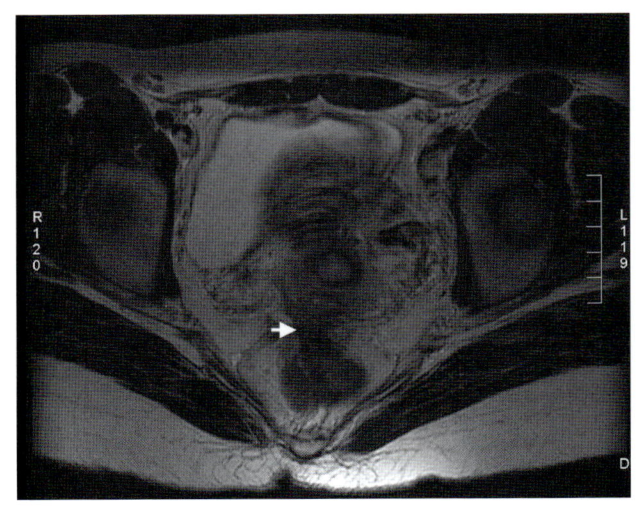

Fig. 2.8 MRI, T_2-weighted imaging, axial plane. Area of endometriosis with prevalent fibrosis (*arrow*), in the rectovaginal septum, with a signal close to that of pelvic muscle

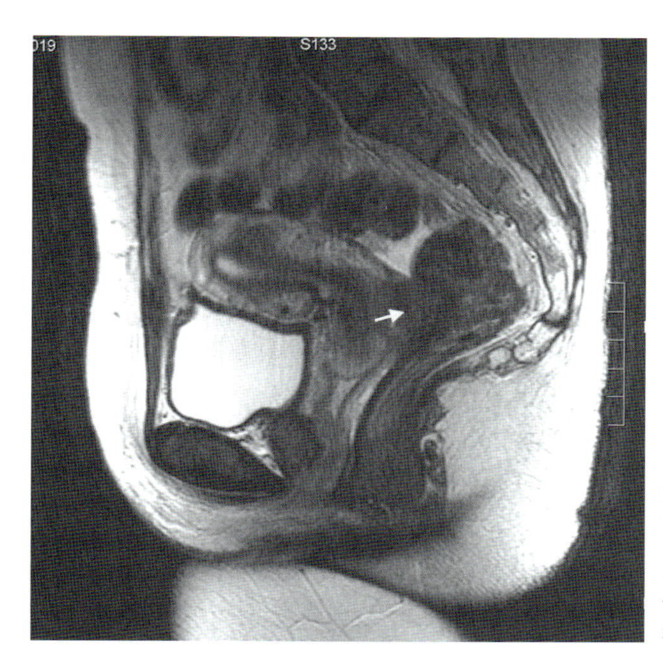

Fig. 2.9 Same case as Fig. 2.8, MRI, T_2-weighted imaging, sagittal plane. Endometriotic nodule invading the anterior rectal wall and posterior fornix (*arrow*)

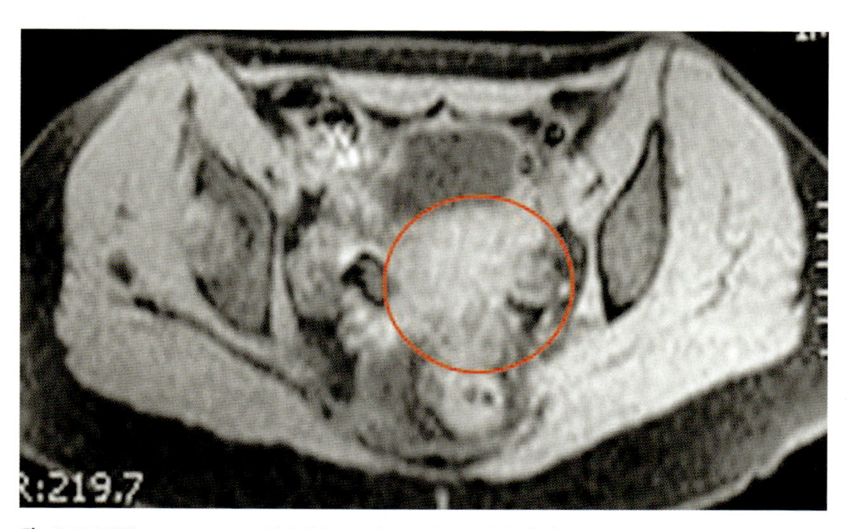

Fig. 2.10 MRI appearance of bladder endometrioma (circled)

native T_1-weighted images without fat suppression, and fat-suppressed T_1-weighted images before and after intravenous injection of gadolinium contrast media (Figs. 2.11 and 2.12).

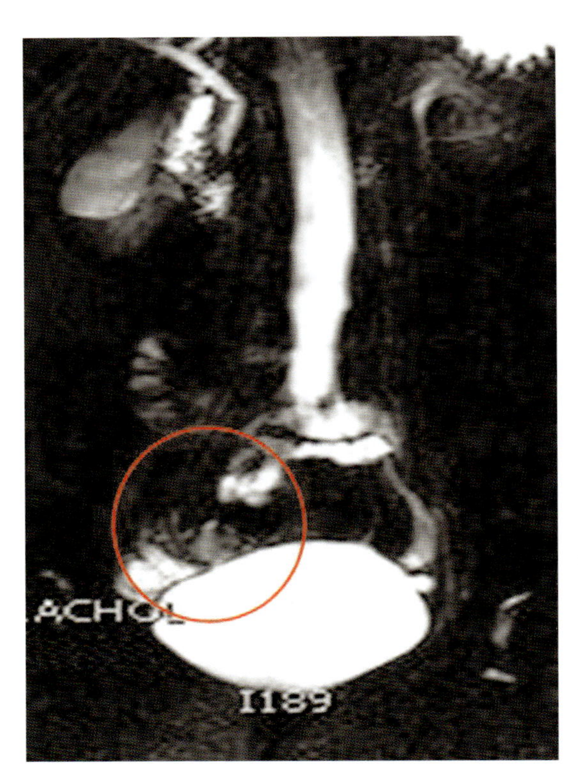

Fig. 2.11 Magnetic resonance urography for ureteral endometrioma (circled). This is a peculiar MRI reconstruction, represented by heavily T_2-weighted sequences. This reconstruction may be useful in detecting ureterohydronephrosis and evaluating other pathology in the abdomen and pelvis

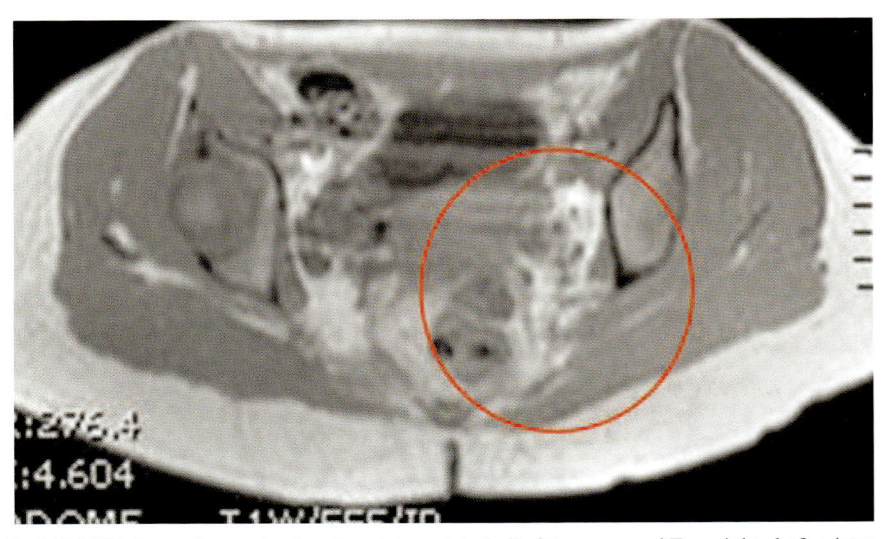

Fig. 2.12 MRI diagnosing ureteral endometrioma (circled); fat-suppressed T_1-weighted after intravenous injection of gadolinium contrast media

In a very recent study by Grasso et al [45], the sensitivity and specificity of MRI in diagnosing deep infiltration of the uterosacral ligament were 69.2% and 94.3% respectively. Posterior vaginal fornix involvement was diagnosed with a sensitivity of 83.3% and specificity of 88.8%. In diagnosing endometriosis of the rectovaginal septum, MRI showed a sensitivity of 76.4% and a specificity of 100%. The sensitivity and specificity of MRI for sigmoid colon involvement were 75% and 100% respectively. The infiltration of ureters was seen with a sensitivity and specificity of 66.6% and 100% and of the bladder with a sensitivity and specificity of 83.3% and 100%.

According to what has been previously reported, different imaging methods are required to effectively assess the disease extent in DIE, which is a multifocal disease. These include TVS, EUS, and MRI. Diagnosis of endometriomas, and vaginal and rectovaginal endometriosis is reliable on ultrasonography. However, in patients with a consistent clinical suspicion of deep pelvic endometriosis, MRI represents an optimal "all-in-one" exam to diagnose and define the exact extent of DIE; as this represents a multifocal disease, it requires an imaging method that is able to cover the entire pelvis to diagnose all possible lesions. High-contrast resolution, multiplanarity, and greater field of view are the main advantages of MRI.

On the other hand, a limitation of MRI is that some intestinal nodules may contain extensive fibrosis [29], which can be viewed as iso-intense to the muscle in both T_1- and T_2-weighted images. Another limitation is the duration of the examination, which may be altered by artefacts due to intestinal peristaltic movements. For this reason, most authors perform an intravenous injection of antispasmodic drug to limit bowel peristalsis. The introduction of an ultrasonographic gel into the vagina to distend the vaginal fornices has also been described.

2.6.9 Colonoscopy

Colonoscopy offers little help in the diagnosis of intestinal endometriosis, because the disease affects the intestinal wall from outside, from the peritoneum, so that lesions are typically subserosal.

In a few patients with large intestinal lesions, colonoscopy may offer the possibility to diagnose an intestinal stenosis or substenosis. The major use of colonoscopy is to histologically distinguish intestinal endometriotic lesions from malignant pathology [29].

2.6.10 Double-contrast Barium Enema

Double-contrast barium enema (DCBE) has been applied in the diagnosis of intestinal DIE. DCBE has the great advantage of being easily reproducible and is also less expensive than EUS and MRI [25]. Like colonoscopy, DCBE also offers little help in the diagnosis of intestinal endometriosis, because lesions are typically subserosal. They appear as an extrinsic mass that compresses the intestinal lumen and may even show a wrinkling of the colon mucosa. This imaging approach only permits definition of the longitudinal extension of that stenosis, but the endoscopic tool cannot pass through this to better define the surgical approach with the colorectal surgeon, and it cannot evaluate its extension through the intestinal wall or its exact distance from the anal sphincter [48].

2.6.11 Computerized Tomography

Computerized tomography (CT) is sometimes proposed as a diagnostic alternative for DIE, because of its importance in localization of endometriotic foci involving the urinary tract. The most important limitation of this technology is the ionizing radiation used. In recent years, CT has been substituted by MRI because of its high accuracy and noninvasiveness (Figs. 2.13 and 2.14).

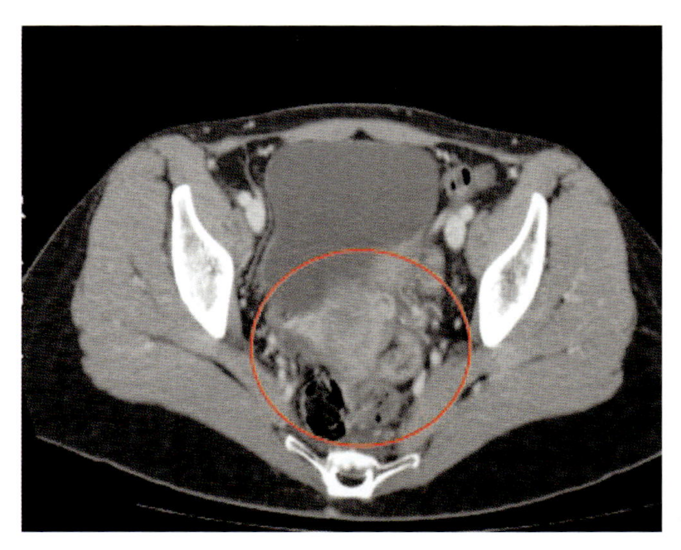

Fig. 2.13 CT image of a large bladder endometrioma (circled)

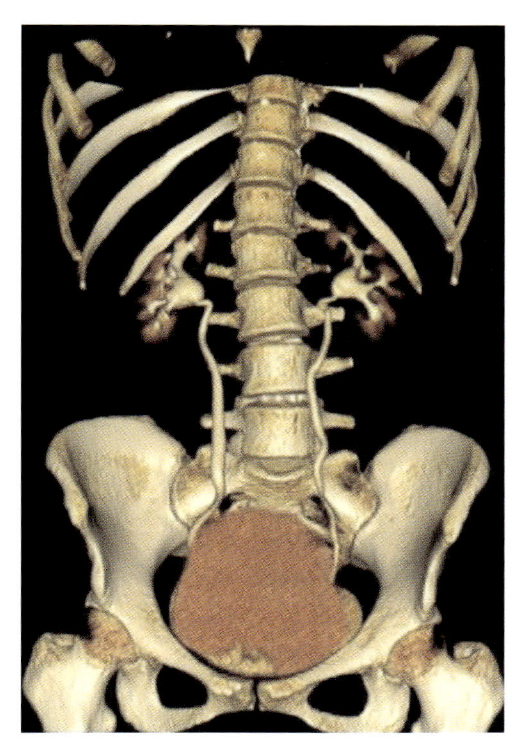

Fig. 2.14 CT three-dimensional reconstruction of the urinary tract, in order to evaluate eventual ureteral involvement by the bladder endometrioma

A new CT technique of computerized, multislice CT enteroclysis requires intestinal preparation, pharmacological hypotonization, and distension of the intestinal lumen by enteroclysis. A study by Biscaldi et al [49] showed a sensitivity of 98.7% and specificity of 100%, with a NPV of 95.7% for identifying women with intestinal endometriosis. It permits an accurate description of the depth and extent of endometriosis in the bowel wall and also permits evaluation of the whole colon, not just its distal tract.

2.6.12 Cystoscopy

Cystoscopy is recommended for all patients with endometriosis and lower urinary tract symptoms or haematuria, since it represents one of the most cost-effective tests [32, 50–52]. The macroscopic appearance of bladder endometrioma lesions may change with the phases of the menstrual cycle; they are often edematous and irregular, with different shapes and colors: blue-red, blue-black, or blue-brown lesions are the most common findings

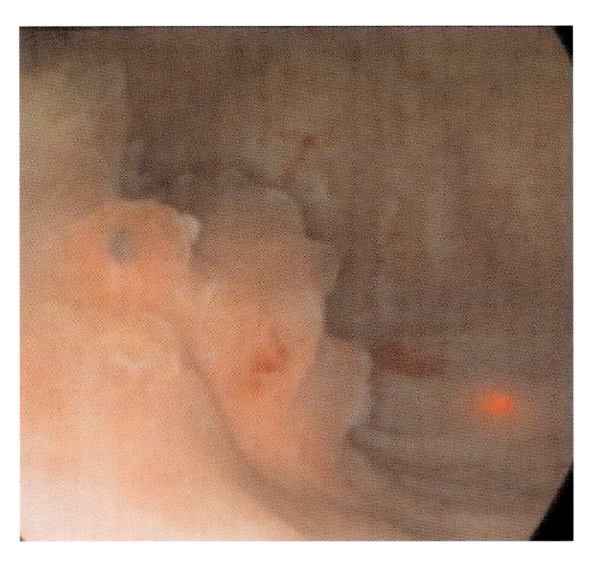

Fig. 2.15 Cystoscopic appearance of bladder endometrioma. The macroscopic appearance of this isolated bladder endometrioma is edematous and irregular, with typical blue-red lesions. The diameter is about 1 cm and the localization is 1.5 cm up to the right ureteral orifice. (Reproduced with permission from www.nezhat.com/images/endo-bladder.jpg)

[16, 53–55] (Fig. 2.15). The areas of bladder endometrioma might be isolated or multifocal, approximately 1 cm in average diameter, and usually located at the dome or at the base. It is fundamental to ascertain the distance between the ureteral orifices and the lower endometriotic margin [54, 56]. Repeat cystoscopy in different phases of the menstrual cycle is recommended, as endometriosis is best diagnosed before and during menstruation. Coupled with biopsy, cystoscopy is the preferred method for visualizing and confirming bladder endometrioma [51]. Moreover, the lesion needs to be differentiated from bladder carcinoma, varices, papillomas, or angiomas [57].

2.6.13 Intravenous Pyelography

Intravenous pyelography (IVP) has been the traditional functional imaging modality used to evaluate women suspected of having ureteral endometriosis [32]. Radiologic findings, including hydroureteronephrosis, narrowing of the pelvic ureter and, rarely, an intraluminal ureteral mass, are judged to be nonspecific for the condition [58]. However, IVP is of value in demonstrating the precise location, extent, and degree of ureteral stenosis, as well as for confirming renal function. Differential diagnosis includes a number of urologic causes of intrinsic or extrinsic ureteral stricture, including primary or metastatic cancer, retroperitoneal lymphadenopathy, and idiopathic retroperitoneal fibrosis. The history is valuable in differentiating endometriosis from strictures due to previous surgery or to trauma, such as stone extraction. Transitional cell carcinoma can be radiologically indistinguishable from ureteral endometriosis, but such tumors are rare in premenopausal women and, unlike endometriosis, typically have an irregular mucosal pattern and are associated with dilatation of the ureter below the lesion. Despite its limitations, IVP, coupled with retrograde pyelography, still remains the most common and valuable test used to assess intrinsic ureteral endometriosis [59].

2.6.14 Ureteroscopy

Ureteroscopy (UR) has been used to diagnose intrinsic ureteral endometriosis [60, 61]. This examination allows both direct observation of the bladder and/or ureteral lesions and provision of specimens for histology by biopsies. It is essential to remember that the macroscopic appearance of the lesions changes with the different phases of the menstrual cycle, analogously to bladder endometrioma. In addition, if the ectopic tissue does not extend beyond the pericystium or ureteral adventitial layer, endoscopy might be useless. Thus, negative endoscopic findings do not necessarily imply the absence of urinary endometriosis.

UR biopsy to establish the diagnosis followed by endoscopic ablation remains a useful, minimally invasive option for some patients with localized ureteral endometrioma [61].

2.7 Conclusions

In conclusion, preoperative instrumental diagnosis of DIE is fundamental to planning the surgical approach. It will be useful to know all the characteristics of the lesion, not merely whether endometriosis is present. Therefore, the number of nodules, whether and how deeply they infiltrate the bowel wall, and their distance from the anal sphincter are important to define the surgical technique (i.e. nodulectomy instead of bowel resection) [62]. Moreover, the operation planning allows the patient to be adequately informed about the surgical risks and the eventual consequences, when obtaining a complete informed consent [63].

Therefore, when a medical treatment option is recommended, TVS examination may be sufficient. From the surgical point of view, the data shown confirm that one advantage of EUS is its ability to determine the distance of colorectal lesions from the anal margins when segmental resection is required, whereas MRI represents an optimal method to diagnose and define the exact extent of DIE, and is able to cover the entire pelvis to diagnose all possible lesions.

Aknowledgments This chapter has been written with the collaboration of F. Di Puppo (Department of Obstetrics and Gynaecology, San Raffaele Scientific Institute, Milan, Italy).

References

1. Hadfield R, Mardon H, Barlow D, Kennedy S. Delay in the diagnosis of endometriosis: a survey of women from the USA and the UK. Hum Reprod 1996;11:878–880
2. Sinaii N, Plumb K, Cotton L et al. Differences in characteristics among 1,000 women with endometriosis based on extent of disease. Fertil Steril 2008;89:538–545
3. Kennedy S, Bergqvist A, Chapron C et al; ESHRE Special Interest Group for Endometriosis and Endometrium Guideline Development Group. ESHRE guideline for the diagnosis and treatment of endometriosis. Hum Reprod 2005;20:2698–2704
4. Seaman HE, Ballard KD, Wright JT, de Vries CS. Endometriosis and its coexistence with irritable bowel syndrome and pelvic inflammatory disease: findings from a national case-control study – part 2. BJOG 2008;115:1392–1396
5. Ballard KD, Seaman HE, de Vries CS, Wright JT. Can symptomatology help in the diagnosis of endometriosis? Findings from a national case-control study – part 1. BJOG 2008; 115:1382–1391
6. Hassa H, Tanir HM, Uray M. Symptom distribution among infertile and fertile endometriosis cases with different stages and localisations. Eur J Obstet Gynecol Reprod Biol 2005;119:82–86
7. Endometriosis GIplSd (Gruppo Italiano per lo Studio dell'endometriosi). Relationship between stage, site and morphological characteristics of pelvic endometriosis and pain. Hum Reprod 2001;16:2668–2671
8. Hurd WW. Criteria that indicate endometriosis is the cause of chronic pelvic pain. Obstet Gynecol 1998;92:1029–1032
9. Porpora MG, Koninckx PR, Piazze J et al. Correlation between endometriosis and pelvic pain. J Am Assoc Gynecol Laparosc 1999;6:429–434
10. Koninckx PR, Meuleman C, Demeyere S et al. Suggestive evidence that pelvic endometriosis is a progressive disease, whereas deeply infiltrating endometriosis is associated with pelvic pain. Fertil Steril 1991;55:759–765
11. Chapron C, Barakat H, Fritel X et al. Presurgical diagnosis of posterior deep infiltrating endometriosis based on a standardized questionnaire. Hum Reprod 2005;20:507–513
12. Berkley KJ, Dmitrieva N, Curtis KS, Papka RE. Innervation of ectopic endometrium in a rat model of endometriosis. Proc Natl Acad Sci U S A 2004;101:11094–11098
13. Tokushige N, Markham R, Russell P, Fraser IS. Nerve fibres in peritoneal endometriosis. Hum Reprod 2006;21:3001–3007

14. Tariverdian N, Theoharides TC, Siedentopf F et al. Neuroendocrine-immune disequilibrium and endometriosis: an interdisciplinary approach. Semin Immunopathol 2007;29:193–210
15. Bulun SE. Endometriosis. Review. N Engl J Med 2009;360:268–279
16. Donnez J, Nisolle M, Squifflet J. Ureteral endometriosis: a complication of rectovaginal endometriotic (adenomyotic) nodules. Fertil Steril 2002;77:32–37
17. Carmignani L, Vercellini P, Spinelli M et al. Pelvic endometriosis and hydroureteronephrosis. Fertil Steril 2010;93:1741–1744
18. Crosignani PG, Vercellini P. Conservative surgery for severe endometriosis: should laparotomy be abandoned definitively? Hum Reprod 1995;10:2412–2418
19. Abrao SM, Gonçalves MO, Antonio Dias J et al. Comparison between clinical examination, transvaginal sonography and magnetic resonance imaging for the diagnosis of deep endometriosis. Hum Reprod 2007;22:3092–3097
20. Marc Bazot, Clarisse Lafont, Roman Rouzier et al. Diagnostic accuracy of physical examination, transvaginal sonography, rectal endoscopic sonography, and magnetic resonance imaging to diagnose deep infiltrating endometriosis. Fertil Steril 2009;92:1825–1833
21. Barbieri RL, Niloff JM, Bast RC Jr et al. Elevated serum concentrations of CA-125 in patients with advanced endometriosis. Fertil Steril 1986;45:630–634
22. Matalliotakis I, Panidis D, Vlassis G et al. Unexpected increase of the CA 19-9 tumour marker in patients with endometriosis. Eur J Gynaecol Oncol 1998;19:498–500
23. Pittaway DE, Fayez JA. The use of CA-125 in the diagnosis and management of endometriosis. Fertil Steril 1986;46:790–795
24. Harada T, Kubota T, Aso T. Usefulness of CA19.9 versus CA125 for the diagnosis of endometriosis. Fertil Steril 2002;78:733–739
25. Somigliana E, Viganò P, Tirelli AS et al. Use of the concomitant serum dosage of CA 125, CA 19-9 and interleukin-6 to detect the presence of endometriosis. Results from a series of reproductive age women undergoing laparoscopic surgery for benign gynaecological conditions. Hum Reprod 2004;19:1871–1876
26. Xavier P, Beires J, Belo L et al. Are we employing the most effective CA 125 and CA 19-9 cut-off values to detect endometriosis? Eur J Obstet Gynecol Reprod Biol 2005;123:254–255
27. Kurdoglu Z, Gursoy R, Kurdoglu M et al. Comparison of the clinical value of CA 19–9 versus CA 125 for the diagnosis of endometriosis. Fertil Steril 2009;92:1761–1763
28. Del Frate C, Girometti R, Pittino M et al. Deep retroperitoneal pelvic endometriosis: MR imaging appearance with laparoscopic correlation. Radiographics 2006;26:1705–1718
29. Bazot M, Detchev R, Cortez A et al. Transvaginal sonography and rectal endoscopic sonography for the assessment of pelvic endometriosis: a preliminary comparison. Hum Reprod 2003;18:1686–1692
30. Bozdech JM. Endoscopic diagnosis of colonic endometriosis. Gastrointest Endosc 1992;38:568–570
31. Chapron C, Dubuisson JB, Pansini V et al. Routine clinical examination is not sufficient for diagnosing and locating deeply infiltrating endometriosis. J Am Assoc Gynecol Laparosc 2002;9:115–119
32. Comiter CV. Endometriosis of the urinary tract. Urol Clin North Am 2002;29:625–635
33. Vercellini P, Meschia M, De Giorgi O et al. Bladder detrusor endometriosis: clinical and pathogenetic implications. J Urol 1996;155:84–86
34. Seracchioli R, Mannini D, Colombo FM et al. Cystoscopy-assisted laparoscopic resection of extramucosal bladder endometriosis. J Endourol 2002;16:663–666
35. Bazot M, Thomassin I, Hourani R et al. Diagnostic accuracy of transvaginal sonography for deep pelvic endometriosis. Ultrasound Obstet Gynecol 2004;24:180–185
36. Carmignani L, Ronchetti A, Amicarelli F et al. Bladder psoas hitch in hydronephrosis due to pelvic endometriosis: outcome of urodynamic parameters. Fertil Steril 2009;92:35–40

37. Roseau G, Dumontier I, Palazzo L et al. Rectosigmoid endometriosis: endoscopic ultrasound features and clinical implications. Endoscopy 2000;32:525–530
38. Bazot M, Thomassin I, Hourani R et al. Diagnostic accuracy of transvaginal sonography for deep pelvic endometriosis. Ultrasound Obstet Gynecol 2004;24:180–185
39. Bazot M, Malzy P, Cortez A et al. Accuracy of transvaginal sonography and rectal endoscopic sonography in the diagnosis of deep infiltrating endometriosis. Ultrasound Obstet Gynecol 2007;30:994–1001
40. Valenzano Menada M, Remorgida V, Abbamonte LH et al. Does transvaginal ultrasonography combined with water-contrast in the rectum aid in the diagnosis of rectovaginal endometriosis infiltrating the bowel? Hum Reprod 2008;23:1069–1075
41. Dessole S, Farina M, Rubattu G et al. Sonovaginography is a new technique for assessing rectovaginal endometriosis. Fertil Steril 2003;79:1023–1027
42. Guerriero S, Ajossa S, Gerada M et al. "Tenderness-guided" transvaginal ultrasonography: a new method for the detection of deep endometriosis in patients with chronic pelvic pain. Fertil Steril 2007;88:1293–1297
43. Vercellini P, Somigliana E, Viganò P et al. Endometriosis: current and future medical therapies. Best Pract Res Clin Obstet Gynaecol 2008;22:275–306
44. Seow KM, Lin YH, Hsieh BC et al. Transvaginal three-dimensional ultrasonography combined with serum CA 125 level for the diagnosis of pelvic adhesions before laparoscopic surgery. J Am Assoc Gynecol Laparosc 2003;10:320–326
45. Grasso RF, Di Giacomo V, Sedati P et al. Diagnosis of deep infiltrating endometriosis: accuracy of magnetic resonance imaging and transvaginal 3D ultrasonography. Abdom Imaging 2009; Nov 19 [Epub ahead of print]
46. Siegelman ES, Outwater E, Wang T, Mitchell DG. Solid pelvic masses caused by endometriosis: MR imaging features. AJR Am J Roentgenol 1994;163:357–361
47. Chapron C, Vieira M, Chopin N et al. Accuracy of rectal endoscopic ultrasonography and magnetic resonance imaging in the diagnosis of rectal involvement for patients presenting with deeply infiltrating endometriosis. Ultrasound Obstet Gynecol 2004;24:175–179
48. Anaf V, El Nakadi I, De Moor V et al. Anatomic significance of a positive barium enema in deep infiltrating endometriosis of the large bowel. World J Surg 2009;33:822–827
49. Biscaldi E, Ferrero S, Fulcheri E et al. Multislice CT enteroclysis in the diagnosis of bowel endometriosis. Eur Radiol 2007;17:211–219
50. Antonelli A, Simeone C, Canossi E et al. Surgical approach to urinary endometriosis: experience on 28 cases. Arch Ital Urol Androl 2006;78:35–38
51. Gustilo-Ashby AM, Paraiso MF. Treatment of urinary tract endometriosis. J Minim Invasive Gynecol 2006;13:559–565
52. Shook TE, Nyberg LM. Endometriosis of the urinary tract. Urology 1988;31:1–6
53. Pastor-Navarro H, Giménez-Bachs JM, Donate-Moreno MJ et al. Update on the diagnosis and treatment of bladder endometriosis. Int Urogynecol J Pelvic Floor Dysfunct 2007;18:949–954
54. Westney OL, Amundsen CL, McGuire EJ. Bladder endometriosis: conservative management. J Urol 2000;163:1814–1817
55. Abeshouse BS, Abeshouse G. Endometriosis of the urinary tract: a review of the literature and a report of four cases of vesical endometriosis. J Int Coll Surg 1960;34:43–63
56. Chapron C, Bourret A, Chopin N et al. Surgery for bladder endometriosis: long-term results and concomitant management of associated posterior deep lesions. Hum Reprod 2010;25: 884–889
57. Granese R, Candiani M, Perino A et al. Bladder endometriosis: laparoscopic treatment and follow-up. Eur J Obstet Gynecol Reprod Biol 2008;140:114–117
58. Pollack HM, Wills JS. Radiographic features of ureteral endometriosis. AJR Am J Roentgenol 1978;131:627–631

59. Yohannes P. Ureteral endometriosis. J Urol 2003;170:20–25
60. Zanetta G, Webb MJ, Segura JW. Ureteral endometriosis diagnosed at ureteroscopy. Obstet Gynecol 1998;91:857–859
61. Generao SE, Keene KD, Das S. Endoscopic diagnosis and management of ureteral endometriosis. J Endourol 2005;19:1177–1179
62. Remorgida V, Ragni N, Ferrero S et al. The involvement of the interstitial Cajal cells and the enteric nervous system in bowel endometriosis. Hum Reprod 2005;20:264–271
63. Remorgida V, Ferrero S, Fulcheri E et al. Bowel endometriosis: presentation, diagnosis, and treatment. Obstet Gynecol Surv 2007;62:461–470

Treatment

3

P. De Nardi, S. Ferrari

Abstract Endocrine pharmacotherapy can be used as a neoadjuvant or adjuvant measure; however, in the majority of symptomatic cases, surgical resection is the treatment of choice for deeply infiltrating endometriosis, to improve pain, quality of life, and possibly fertility.

The goal should be to achieve the complete treatment of all endometriotic lesions by a single operation. Since more complex cases require resection of the intestinal wall and/or bladder or ureter, the expertise and cooperation of different specialists, namely colorectal and urologic surgeons, is warranted.

Many retrospective studies have demonstrated the beneficial effect of conservative surgery for pain symptoms; however, few studies have reported long-term follow-up data

In the case of rectal or rectosigmoid involvement, a formal bowel resection, rather than partial excision, is most often preferable, despite the fact that it entails a higher risk of intraoperative and postoperative complications. In cases of bladder endometriosis, transurethral resection, partial cystectomy, or combined operations can be performed, whereas, when the ureter is involved, ureterolysis, ureterostomy, and ureteral reimplantation are carried out.

Laparoscopic and laparotomic resections achieve the same

P. De Nardi (✉)
Department of Surgery, San Raffaele Scientific Institute, Milan, Italy

results in terms of symptom control, although the complexity of the disease or extensive involvement of extragenital organs sometimes requires laparotomy, or carries a high risk of conversion.

Data on reoperation for rectovaginal endometriosis and repetitive conservative surgery are scant.

Keywords Laparoscopy • Resection • Bowel • Ureter • Rectovaginal • Complications • Recurrence • Follow-up

3.1 Medical Therapy

Once the diagnosis of endometriosis has been histologically confirmed, endocrine pharmacotherapy can be used as a neoadjuvant or adjuvant measure, as well as for treatment of recurrences. Surgeons generally do not favor neoadjuvant endocrine pharmacotherapy because of its unfavorable effect on tissue surfaces. In cases of extensive endometriosis, and particularly in deeply infiltrating endometriosis (DIE), a R0 resection can only rarely be achieved. It therefore makes sense to give adjuvant endocrine pharmacotherapy with the goal of transient therapeutic amenorrhea. The following options are available at present:

a. progestagens;
b. oral contraceptives;
c. gonadotropin-releasing hormone (GnRH) analogs;
d. pain therapy;
e. combinations of the above;
f. experimental treatment approaches.

Progestagens effect a secretory transformation of the endometrium after previous exposure to estrogens.

Oral contraceptives (when used off-label for this indication) bring about a so-called pseudopregnancy regimen. Their well-known side effects, which vary in frequency from one preparation to another, include breakthrough bleeding, nausea, headache, and an elevated risk of venous thromboembolism, as well as loss of libido, cutaneous reactions, and sodium and fluid retention, leading to weight gain, breast tenderness, and a rise in blood pressure. Generally, however, oral contraceptives are very well tolerated.

The goal of treatment is suppression of menses (therapeutic amenorrhea). If breakthrough bleeding occurs, the patient can take one oral contraceptive tablet twice a day for as long as smear bleeding persists and for one day afterwards, and then return to a single tablet per day. It is important for the patient to be properly informed.

GnRH analogs bring about a "functional oophorectomy", that is, a state of pharmacologically induced hypogonadotropic hypogonadism. This, in turn, causes well-recognized side effects such as hot flashes and perspiration (80% to 90%), sleep disturbance (60% to 90%), vaginal dryness (30%), headache (20% to 30%), mood changes (depressive mood change because of estrogen withdrawal, more than 10%), osteopenia, loss of libido (more than 30%), and weight gain (about 15%).

3.1.1 Combined Treatment Approaches (Pharmacotherapy and Pain Therapy)

In addition to surgery and pharmacotherapy, complementary treatments, whose efficacy has not been documented by scientific evidence, can be used. Women whose quality of life is impaired by cyclic or chronic pain need treatment in order to achieve a pain-free state with a better quality of life and an improved ability to engage in productive activities. In a specialized endometriosis center, the patient's individual situation can be stabilized or improved through a team effort, with the active participation of the patient herself, her treating gynecologist, the surgeon, the pain specialist, and the psychotherapist. Before treatment, these women's problems are often severe enough to cause the loss of a job or of a life partner.

3.1.2 Experimental Treatment Approaches

Endometriosis cells manifest properties such as invasiveness, migration, metastasis, angiogenesis, and neurogenesis that call to mind similar properties of malignant tumors. Their responsiveness to cytokines, tumor necrosis factor (TNF-α), cyclooxygenase-2 (COX-2), oxytocin, and aromatase is currently being exploited in an attempt to devise new methods for diagnosis and treatment [1–4]. Although a combination of aromatase inhibitors with progestagens or GnRH analogs has been proven to be effective, the practicality of this form of treatment is currently limited by both its side effects and its cost [2].

3.2 Surgery

There is a general consensus that surgical resection is the treatment of choice for deep pelvic infiltration (DIE) [5, 6]. Surgery should be considered after a careful and complete evaluation of the patient and should be based on the extent of disease, severity of symptoms, and desire for pregnancy [7]. Consequently, the aim should be to improve pain, quality of life, and possibly fertility. These goals should preferably be achieved by a single operation, allowing complete treatment of all endometriotic lesions. As a consequence, the cooperation of different specialists is warranted. Since the diagnosis of DIE has a wide range of anatomical scenarios, therapeutic planning is extremely flexible and should be adapted to the individual case.

Surgery is defined as conservative when the ability to conceive is retained. There is no consensus about the possible improvement of fertility with surgery, since in most cases it seems as effective as medical treatment; however, surgical ablation of endometriotic tissue seems superior in patients with the most severe forms of endometriosis. Many studies demonstrate a long-lasting improvement of pain symptoms by the application of conservative surgical treatment, with symptomatic recurrence in approximately one-quarter of patients.

In asymptomatic patients with endometriotic nodules located in the rectovaginal septum, Fedele et al demonstrated disease progression or appearance of specific symptoms in less than 10% of women, during a 5-year observational period. Although the study was conducted in a limited number of patients, the authors suggest that if the patient is asymptomatic, the disease does not require specific treatment, especially surgery, and recommend that watchful waiting is preferable [8].

However, in the majority of symptomatic cases surgery seems to be the only effective treatment. When surgical treatment is chosen and the best possible mapping obtained by imaging techniques, some other parameters should be considered:

- previous surgical procedures the patient has undergone;
- the presence and diffusion of adherences;
- the presence, location, size, and distance from the anal margin of digestive involvement, as well as the depth of bowel-wall infiltration;
- the presence and location of ureter or bladder involvement [9].

In simpler cases, excision of the endometriotic nodule is feasible and is considered the most appropriate solution. Nevertheless, most complex cases require resection of the intestinal wall and/or bladder or ureter [6].

Laparoscopic resection is now considered feasible and safe [10] (Figs. 3.1 and 3.2); however, extensive involvement of extragenital organs, such as the bladder and bowel, sometimes requires laparotomy [11, 12].

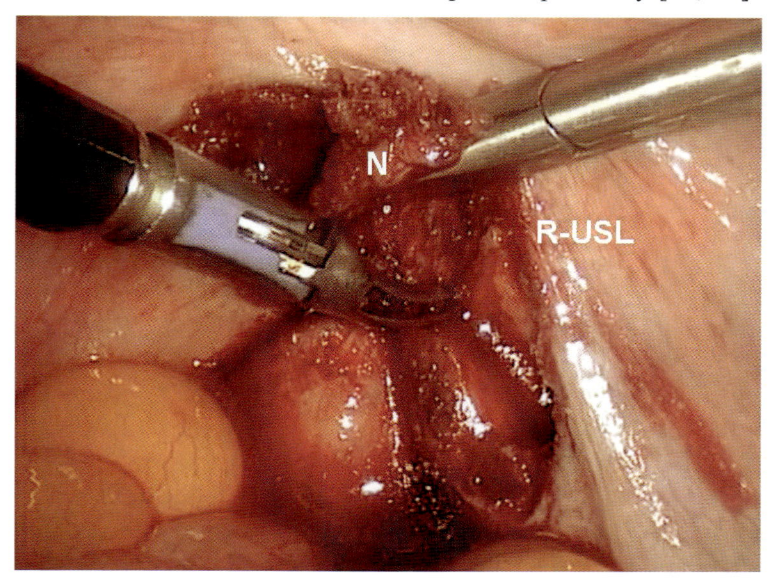

Fig. 3.1 Laparoscopic excision of endometriotic nodule (*N*) on the right uterosacral ligament (*R-USL*)

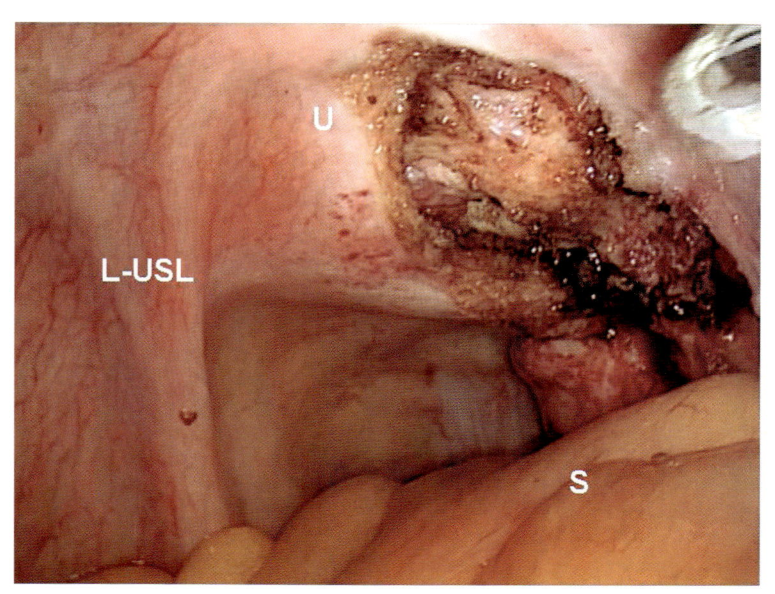

Fig. 3.2 The operating field at the end of operation. *L-USL*, left uterosacral ligament; *S*, sigmoid colon; *U*, uterus

In any event, the surgical treatment of DIE is a real challenge for the gynecologic surgeon and requires the expertise and cooperation of different specialists, namely colorectal and urologic surgeons [13, 14].

In addition to resection, two techniques, uterosacral nerve ablation and presacral neurectomy, have been proposed to treat specific symptoms and to improve antalgic results [15].

3.2.1 Laparoscopic Uterosacral Nerve Ablation

Laparoscopic uterosacral nerve ablation (LUNA) involves bilateral transection of the uterosacral ligaments close to their insertion into the cervix. The procedure interrupts pelvic afferent sensory nerve fibers to the uterus. In 1955 Doyle described transection of the uterosacral nerves from the vagina: this technique was effective for dysmenorrhea [16]. Since then several uncontrolled studies have supported the use of LUNA for both primary and secondary dysmenorrhea. The best results have been obtained in patients with midline referred pain. Despite its rationale, the results remain controversial: according to a Cochrane meta-analysis, the addition of LUNA was not shown to improve pelvic pain [17]. Moreover, the recurrence of pain after 1 year is as high as 50%. Complications are limited and lower than for presacral neuronectomy, although postoperative bleeding and ureteral damage have been reported; there have also been isolated case reports of uterine prolapse and bladder dysfunction. Some authors propose that this procedure should be routinely included when performing surgery for DIE. Johnson and coworkers reported the effectiveness of LUNA for chronic pelvic pain in the absence of endometriosis, but at present there is insufficient evidence of the effectiveness of adding LUNA to laparoscopic surgical removal of endometriosis [18–20].

3.2.2 Presacral Neurectomy

This procedure consists of disruption of the hypogastric plexus. A small number of randomized controlled trials (RCTs) have examined the efficacy of presacral neurectomy (PN) in addition to conservative surgery, with rather inconsistent results. A recent randomized trial has supported the effectiveness of laparoscopic PN for severe dysmenorrhea related to endometriosis. Women who complain of predominantly midline-hypogastric pain seem to be the best candidates for this intervention.

The procedure requires skill and experience. Particular attention has to be paid to the ureters and major and mid-sacral vessels, since severe hemorrhagic complications, including one fatal case, have been reported. Since the procedure involves transection of a greater number of nerve fibers than LUNA, side effects are not negligible, and should be more rigorously assessed. Adverse side effects include, in particular, constipation, bladder dysfunction, and painless labor [21–23].

3.2.3 Deep Pelvic Infiltration of the Rectovaginal Septum without Intestinal Involvement

There is consensus in the literature that, in symptomatic patients, surgical resection is the best treatment for this form of endometriosis. Many authors agree that laparoscopic or laparoscopy-assisted resection is preferable in DIE involving the rectovaginal septum. Nevertheless, if radical resection cannot be achieved, laparotomy should be preferred to incomplete laparoscopic resection. Many studies show significant pain relief or control with conservative surgery. Dysmenorrhea, dyspareunia, and chronic pelvic pain improve in 60–92%, 70–100%, and 60–93% respectively, while pain recurs in approximately 20% of cases [24–26].

3.2.3.1 Surgical Technique

Even if rectal invasion is not suspected, mechanical bowel preparation should be undertaken. Both a transvaginal and laparoscopic technique are usually employed. Complete separation of the rectovaginal space is accomplished with the help of a probe placed into the vagina and the rectum to improve the exposure and resection of the lesions. The mobilization starts from the right and left pararectal spaces towards the midline; the first step is to free the nodule from the rectal wall; careful dissection with scissors, or a monopolar or harmonic scalpel, is carried out to identify a cleavage plane between the nodules and the anterior wall of the rectum. Secondly, the nodule is dissected from the uterosacral ligaments. At this point, the nodule can be left attached to the posterior wall of the vagina, and exeresis of the lesion is completed by the vaginal route. In other cases, the nodule is dissected from the posterior wall of the vagina and fornix. After removal of the specimen, the rectum is checked by hydropneumatic testing, to rule out possible lesions. Both the ureters should be identified and their integrity verified.

There is still debate on the best surgical technique in terms of feasibility and long-term results. Angioni et al proposed routine excision of the posterior vagina fornix adjacent to the nodule, even if a macroscopic infiltration was not present [26]. They studied 31 women with DIE of the cul-de-sac, and retrocervical and rectovaginal septum without intestinal involvement, in which partial removal of the vagina was accomplished with the aim of preventing recurrence or disease progression. In 10% of cases, microscopic involvement was documented by histopathological analysis. The authors did not observe any recurrence after 5 years' follow-up. This approach prolongs the duration of operation but allows removal of undetected implants [26]. Chapron et al also prefer to remove the infiltrated posterior vaginal wall together with the endometriotic nodule, via the vagina [27]. Fedele and coworkers treated similar cases without removal of vaginal tissue, and documented 28% disease recurrence within 3 years [28].

3.2.4 Deep Infiltrating Endometriosis with Rectal or Rectosigmoid Involvement

Endometriosis may affect the bowel in 3% to 37% of all cases of the disease, and in 90% of these cases the rectum, sigmoid, or both are involved [29, 30]. This form of DIE is considered the most severe, and represents one of the most complex problems in the management of this disease.

Surgery is acknowledged to be very challenging, and the degree of radical excision should always be balanced with the risk of complications. However, it is frequently the case that these risks are preferable to the symptoms of incapacitating pain. The main indications for surgery are acute or chronic intestinal obstruction or doubtful diagnosis with suspicion of bowel malignancy [31, 32]. In all other cases, the choice of surgical treatment in patients with DIE and bowel invasion is difficult, and candidates should be fully informed about the risks of all possible complications. Women who complain of dyspareunia, dysmenorrhea, pain at defecation, and nonmenstrual pelvic pain related to pelvic endometriosis, with poor response to medical treatment, are considered the best candidates for resection [33]. On the other hand, some authors suggest that symptoms like pain on bowel movement, lower back pain, and asthenia may not respond so well to surgical resection and, in absence of other symptoms, would contraindicate extensive surgery [34].

One feature of DIE infiltrating the bowel wall is that even though the activity of the disease may be controlled by medical treatment, regression of the nodule in the muscular tissue will eventually cause fibrosis and scar tissue that result in persistence or even worsening of intestinal symptoms [14].

Once surgery has been planned, three different options can be chosen: superficial excision, full disc excision, or formal bowel resection. The choice is based mainly on the extent of bowel involvement; however, the optimal treatment is not yet established.

Superficial lesions involving only the serosa can be "shaved off" using scissors. Diathermy may cause delayed postoperative fistula due to thermal damage to the bowel wall, and therefore requires caution. Carbon dioxide laser should be used at low power [35]. Superficial excision has the advantage of preventing intestinal opening; however, it carries the risk of possible microperforation with subsequent pelvic sepsis; hydropneumatic testing should be performed to detect occult leak intraoperatively. Supporters of the "shaving technique" claim that a more conservative approach preserves organs, nerves, and vascular supply, with fewer postoperative complications and higher pregnancy rates [36]. Donnez and Squifflet [37] proposed the shaving technique also for patients with nodules infiltrating the muscularis layer of the rectum, with suturing of the muscularis defect after removal of the nodule; they conducted a prospective study on 500 women with rectovaginal nodules, measuring 2–6 cm, who underwent laparoscopic nodule dissection from the posterior vaginal fornix, the rectal wall, and the uterosacral ligaments. They reported 1.4% intraoperative rectal perforations, which were all immediately repaired laparoscopically. After a median follow-up of 3 years, 57% of women who wished to conceive became pregnant. Pain recurrence was observed in 3.6%.

When invasion of the bowel wall is present, a full-thickness disc excision can be used. After removal of the nodule, the bowel wall is sutured in a single or double layer [38]. Two stay sutures are placed to each side of the defect, and the lumen is then closed transversely to prevent bowel stenosis; we prefer two layers of interrupted stitches. Another technique has been described for resection of deep, low rectal nodules that are no larger than 2 cm: the excision is accomplished by a circular stapler inserted transanally [39–41].

The decision to perform disc excision or bowel resection is generally made case by case, since no guidelines exist on whether to perform a nodulectomy rather than resection. The size and depth of infiltration both play a role, and most authors agree that planned bowel resection is only carried out if invasion involves more than 50% of the bowel circumference, in the case of multiple nodules, or for a single nodule that is larger than 3 cm [42]. However, a study by Remorgida et al demonstrated that full-thickness disc excision led to incomplete disease removal in more than 40% of cases. In fact, foci of endometriosis are found in the bowel wall adjacent to the nodulectomy, with macroscopically clear margins [43]. The hypothesis is that the endometriotic nodules microscopically infiltrate the large bowel wall along the nerves, as shown by Anaf et al [44]; therefore, lesions can be found at a distance from the principal nodules. Abrão and coworkers studied 45 cases of rectal endometriosis and found multiple lesions in 42.2% of cases, and mucosa or submucosa involvement in 64% of cases [45]; moreover, in 90% of these, more than 40% of the rectosigmoid circumference was involved; removal of these lesions with such a large percentage of circumferential wall involvement may result in significant stenosis of the bowel lumen [45]. Kavallaris et al [46] carried out histopathological assessment for rectovaginal endometriosis, of tissue sections from resected bowel, taken every 2 cm from the main lesion, and found multifocal (secondary lesions less than 2 cm from the principal lesion) and multicentric (secondary lesions more than 2 cm from the principal lesion) disease in 62% and 38% of the specimens respectively. Finally, Roman confirmed that active glandular endometrial foci are likely to be missed by single nodule excision [47]. From these studies it seems that it is nearly impossible to macroscopically assess the extent of endometriotic lesions inside the bowel wall, and that secondary lesions can be found even at considerable distance from the main endometriotic nodule. Brouwer and Woods evaluated the recurrence after the three procedures and found recurrence rates of 22%, 5%, and 2% after dissection of the nodule off the rectal wall, disk excision, and rectal resection respectively [13]. In our experience, for more radical surgery, a formal bowel resection rather than a partial excision is most often preferable.

On the other hand, there are several other teams that prefer to perform nodule excision, because of the higher morbidity and the less satisfactory functional results of colorectal resection [37]. As an example, Roman and coworkers mainly performed colorectal resection before 2007, with systematic resection of the posterior vaginal fornix, with the aim of achieving complete removal of the disease. However, after 2007, they considered a nodule excision associated with prolonged postoperative treatment with GnRH. They therefore compared digestive and urinary symptoms in the two groups after a minimum follow-up of 12 months [48]. With all the limitation of a retrospective study and of the small sample size, they found no difference in postoperative pelvic pain in the two groups; women were more likely to suffer from an increase in the daily number of stools, constipation, and urinary dysfunction following colorectal resection. They concluded that the use of prolonged GnRH after nodulectomy is as effective as more extensive surgery [48]. Busacca on the other hand did not find any significative advantage in relation to pain recurrence by employing GnRH postoperatively; recurrence was 23% versus 29% after 18 months [49].

Unfortunately, a study comparing the risk of recurrence after nodule excision and colorectal resection would require several hundred patients with several years follow-up.

3.2.4.1 Surgical Technique: Laparoscopic Bowel Resection

Bowel preparation is carried out the day before operation by intestinal washout with an iso-osmotic solution (2 l). Antibiotic prophylaxis with a single dose of cefotetan (2 g intravenously) is administered during the induction of anesthesia, and a second dose of the same antibiotic is administered if surgery lasts more than 4 h. Deep vein thrombosis prophylaxis is carried out with low molecular weight heparin (3000 IU/day). A multidisciplinary team of gynecologic and colorectal, and sometimes urologic, surgeons is involved.

Pneumoperitoneum is established with an open technique and maintained between 10 and 12 mmHg. Three operative trocars are introduced: a 15 mm trocar in the right pararectal, and 12 mm trocars in the right iliac fossa and median suprapubic area; a fourth 5 mm trocar is inserted in the left iliac fossa when needed. After exploration of the abdominal cavity to evaluate the extent of disease and note all associated lesions, the left colon and rectum are released. After left colon mobilization, the pelvic endometriotic tissue is approached by mobilization of endometriotic lesions including the uterosacral ligaments and pouch of Douglas. Dissection within the rectovaginal septum is facilitated by introducing a probe into the vagina and/or rectum, to better evaluate the area of infiltration and help separate the two organs. The inferior dissection is continued until normal yellow fat is encountered under the nodule. During preparation, a nerve-sparing technique and visualization of both ureters should be used. Once the dissection has been completed, the rectum is freed from the posterior vaginal wall and then divided with an endoscopic surgical stapler, under the endometriotic tissue. Therefore, our goal is to remove, "en bloc", all the endometriotic implants along with the involved bowel.

Treatment of associated lesions is performed next. A 5–7 cm incision is made in the left lower quadrant to allow the colorectum to be exteriorized and resected. After positioning the anvil of the circular stapler, the incision is closed and the pneumoperitoneum re-established; a mechanical double-stapled anastomosis is then fashioned intracorporeally. In exceptional cases, with a very low nodule in the rectovaginal septum, a hand-sewn anastomosis is performed transanally. A drain is then placed in the pelvis. An omentoplasty is finally performed, particularly when rectal anastomosis is associated with vaginal wall repair (Figs. 3.3–3.8).

The specimen containing the rectum can be also resected transanally, as described by Nezhat et al [50], or transvaginally as Redwine and coworkers prefer, through a posterior colpotomy [51]. The vagina can be closed transvaginally or laparoscopically.

However, resection of the rectum through the abdomen, by either laparotomy or laparoscopy has, in our opinion, several advantages over the transanal and transvaginal route: it protects the sphincters and distal rectum from potential trauma and avoids juxtapositioning of vaginal and rectal sutures which potentially carries a higher risk of rectovaginal fistula formation.

Many retrospective studies have demonstrated the beneficial effect of conservative surgery for pain symptoms in 60–100% of patients [13, 31, 33, 52, 53], with around 20% of pain recurrence after 36 months [28].

Redwine and Wright examined preoperative and postoperative symptoms in 67 women who underwent conservative laparoscopic excision of rectovaginal endometriosis associated with complete obliteration of the posterior

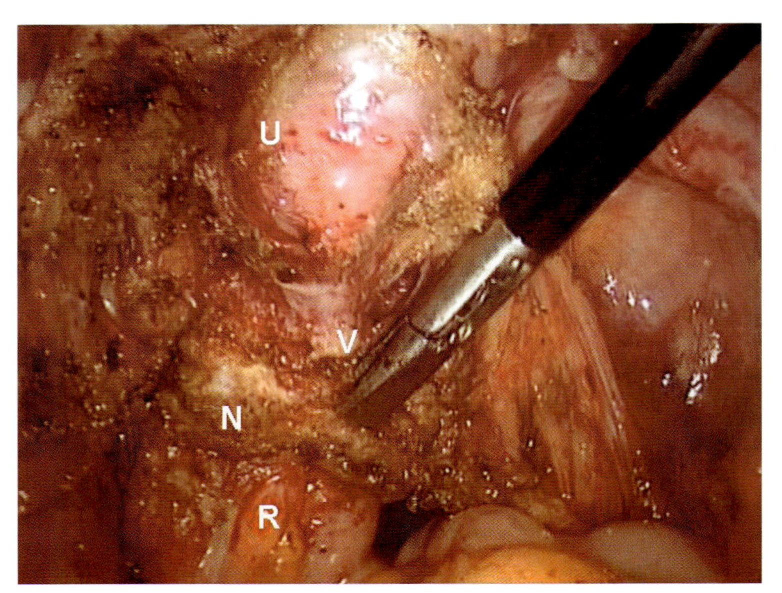

Fig. 3.3 Laparoscopic rectal resection of endometriotic nodule (*N*) in the subperitoneal space of the pouch of Douglas. The rectovaginal space, under the uterus (*U*), is being opened: the nodule invades the anterior rectal wall (*R*) and the posterior vaginal fornix (*V*)

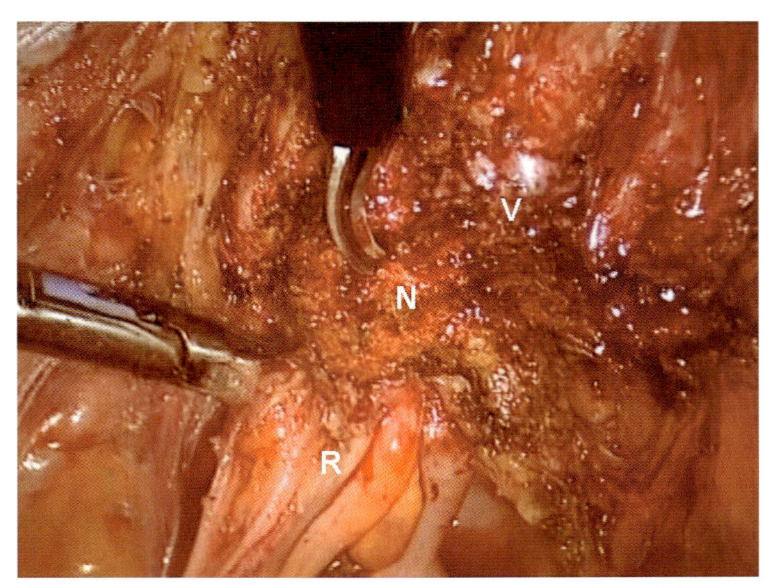

Fig. 3.4 The nodule is dissected from the vagina (*V*). *N*, endometriotic nodule; *R*, anterior rectal wall

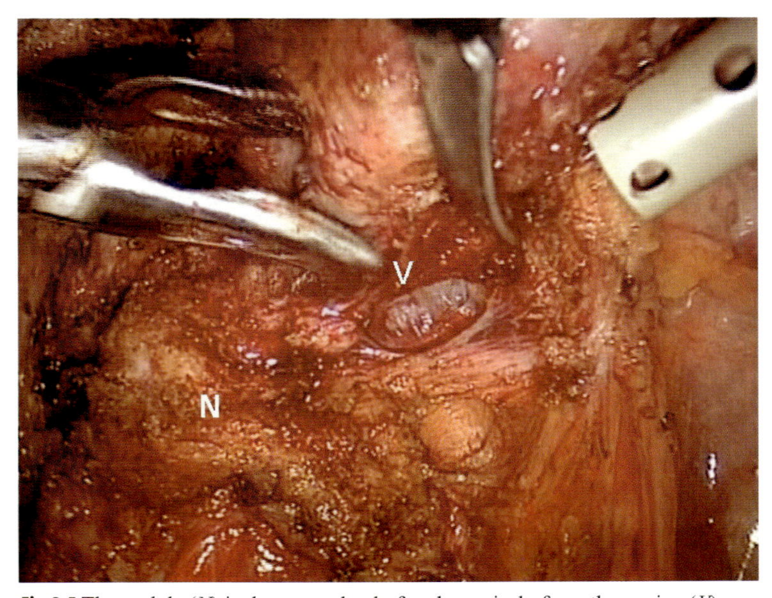

Fig. 3.5 The nodule (*N*) is then completely freed anteriorly from the vagina (*V*)

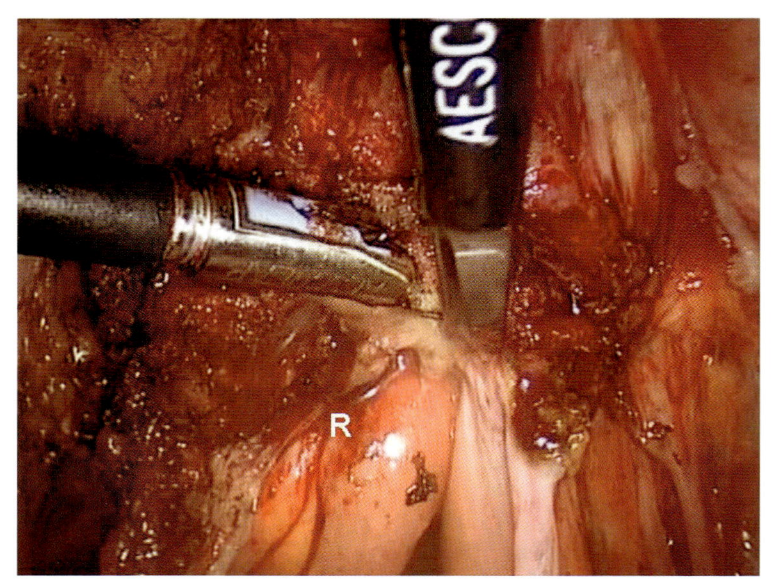

Fig. 3.6 The dissection continues below the lower edge of the nodule and the rectum (*R*) is prepared for the anastomosis

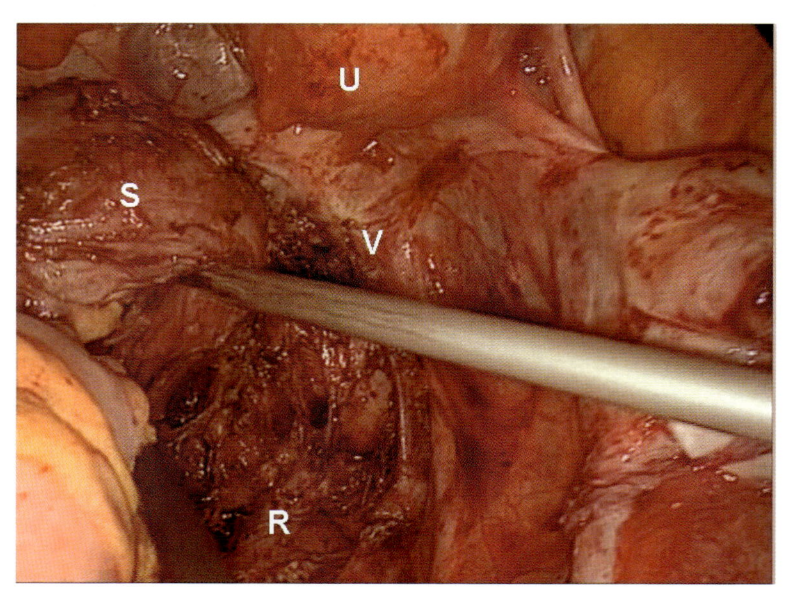

Fig. 3.7 The rectum (*R*) has been resected under the endometriotic nodule. The sigmoid colon (*S*) has been prepared for the anastomosis. *U*, uterus; *V*, vagina

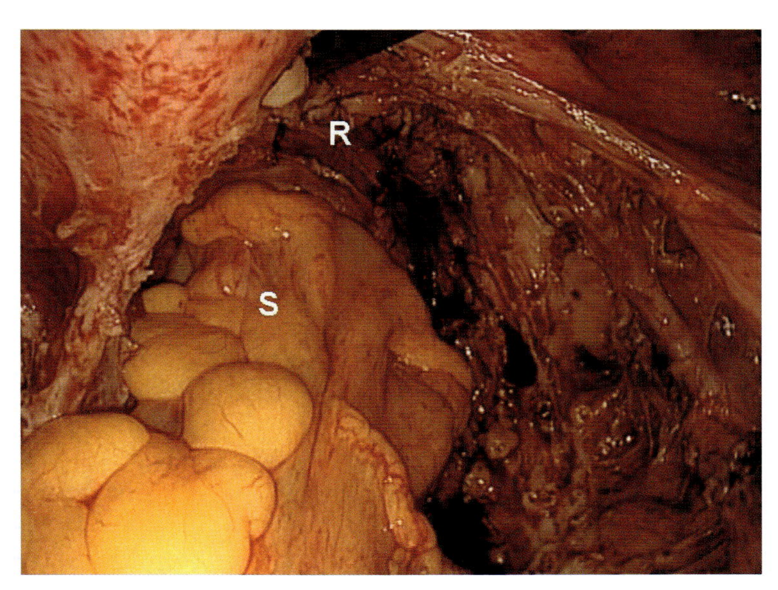

Fig. 3.8 Pelvic floor after completion of the anastomosis between the rectal stump (*R*) and the sigmoid colon (*S*)

cul-de-sac [24]. Irrespective of the procedure performed in the rectum (none, nodulectomy, rectal resection), an improvement of all examined symptoms was found: nonmenstrual pelvic pain improved in 78%, dyspareunia in 66%, and dysmenorrhea in 68%; moreover, several intestinal symptoms, such as cramping, diarrhea, constipation, and painful bowel movements all improved postoperatively [24].

Thomassin et al compared the preoperative and postoperative symptoms intensity score in 27 patients who underwent colorectal resection, and found that resection improved some symptoms but not others; in fact they reported a significant improvement in dysmenorrhea, dyspareunia, pain at defecation, and nonmenstrual pelvic pain; in contrast, no improvement was observed in lower back pain and asthenia [33]. On the other hand, Darai et al reported improvement of all symptoms evaluated, including lower back pain, pain at bowel movement, and asthenia [54].

Fedele et al [28] examined the recurrence of pain symptoms in 83 patients, 30 of whom underwent bowel resection at 36 months' follow-up. They found 28% recurrence of symptoms and clinical evidence of recurrence in 34% of patients. Interestingly, the patients who underwent bowel resection had less chance of suffering recurrence, thus suggesting that more radical surgery had been carried out in this group of patients.

Very few authors have studied factors that correlate with postoperative recurrence. Fedele et al identified younger age and previous surgery for DIE, while the occurrence of a pregnancy decreased the incidence of pain relapse [28]. Other authors emphasize the protective role of pregnancy against pain recurrence. The increased risk of recurrence in younger women is also underlined by Fleish et al in their retrospective study on 23 women [52]. Seracchioli and coworkers described medium term follow-up in women undergoing laparoscopic retosigmoid resection. They found no clinical recurrence after 3 years' follow-up and reported improvement of diarrhea, bleeding, and constipation [55].

A small number of studies have reported long-term follow-up data after conservative surgery. Busacca et al [56] evaluated the probability of recurrence over a 20-year period. They found 30.6% and 43.4% after 4 and 8 years respectively. No difference between laparoscopic and laparotomic resection was found.

Many studies have demonstrated that laparoscopic and laparotomic rectosigmoid resection achieve the same results in terms of pain control. However, these studies are heterogeneous and difficult to compare. The first case of laparoscopic sigmoid resection for endometriosis was reported by Redwine and Sharpe in 1991 [57]. Since then, many papers have reported the results of colorectal resection, with a wide range of complications [29, 34, 54, 58–61]. No prospective randomized studies have compared laparotomic and laparoscopic procedures in terms of operative time and complications, and only one randomized trial has compared open and laparoscopically assisted colorectal resection. In a large series of 436 laparoscopic bowel resections Ruffo et al reported two cases (0.4%) of accidental bowel perforations, distant from the anastomotic site, possibly due to unrecognized intraoperative lesions. These complications seem to be specific to the laparoscopic approach and were treated by re-laparoscopy and colostomy [62]. Two series have compared the results in terms of postoperative pregnancy rate: Fayez and Collazo found that laparoscopy achieved better results [63], while Crosignani et al found a trend towards laparotomy, although it was not significant [64]. Some authors consider the laparotomic approach to be safer and more radical, and suggest that laparotomy should be routinely chosen in all cases in which there is proven rectosigmoid involvement. On the other hand, other authors, mainly colorectal surgeons, consider laparoscopic resection as first-line treatment. The only randomized study, by Darai et al [65], compared open to laparoscopically assisted colorectal resection, in two groups of 26 patients, focusing on complications, symptoms, quality of life, and fertility. The laparoscopically assisted group showed a faster postoperative recovery and fewer complications; symptom relief and quality of life were similar in both groups, with a significant improvement of digestive, gynecological, and general symptoms. Finally, the pregnancy rate was higher in the laparoscopic group [65].

The risk of conversion can be as high as 20% and depends on the experience and skills of the surgeons, body mass index of the patient, intraoperative complications, difficulty of dissection for adhesion, or previous surgical operations, particularly when ureteral involvement is found. The main reasons for conversion are intraoperative complications such as bleeding, or damage to the bladder, ureter, or colon; malfunctioning of the surgical stapler has been also reported [14, 66, 67]. Cases of advanced endometriosis with severe adhesion have a higher risk of intraoperative complications: for these reasons, some authors suggest that patients with these features may not be good candidates for laparoscopic surgery [68]. Duepree et al reported 16.7% intraoperative complications, leading to conversion in 7.8% of cases [58], while Redwine and Wright reported no intraoperative complications in 84 women [24]. Darai et al reported 10% conversion for difficult dissection due to severe adhesion or ureteral involvement, and malfunctioning of the circular stapler [54].

In conclusion, serious concerns persist about the suitability and safety of laparoscopic colorectal resections in patients with deep pelvic endometriosis. In our opinion, laparoscopy, compared with an open technique, seems to achieve the same outcome in terms of improvement of symptoms and quality of life, with lower surgical trauma and possibly fewer complications. Moreover, better visualization of the deep pelvic structures may improve the accuracy of the dissection. However, the laparoscopic approach is time consuming, since longer operative time has been reported [68]. As an example, a mean operative time of 6 h with a duration of 13 h has been reported by Marpeau [59].

Irrespective of the technique of bowel resection, early postoperative complications of bowel resection include: anastomotic dehiscence, rectovaginal fistula, pelvic abscess, and bleeding. Most of these require surgical management [54, 66, 69, 70].

Dehiscence of the colon or rectal anastomosis is reported to be between 1% and 13%. This complication seems more frequent the lower the anastomosis, and the problem is particularly relevant when the anastomosis is below 7 cm from the anal verge. This event requires surgical revision with suture of the anastomosis or resection and reconstruction of the anastomosis and a protective stoma [70].

Rectovaginal fistula is reported to be between 0% and 8.4%. This is a particularly serious complication, since in most cases it requires colostomy. Darai et al reported two cases of rectovaginal fistula due to necrosis of the vaginal fornix, possibly as a result of extensive electrocoagulation [54]. This further supports the use of scissors or an ultrasound system with limited thermal diffusion. When vaginal suture is close to the rectal anastomosis, it is advisable to bring an omental flap between the vagina and the anastomosis to prevent such complication.

Urinary complications are usually associated with extensive involvement of the uterosacral ligaments, with consequent removal of anatomic structures involved in bladder innervation, often combined with extensive rectal resection. Complications include dysuria in 14% and transient urinary retention in 7%; the latter serious complication requires self-catheterization and is generally reversible within 2 weeks to 6 months [33]. Dubernard et al studied urinary complications of surgery in detail, in 58 patients with colorectal involvement of DIE. Almost all the patients reported significant urinary complications, consisting of hesitancy, straining to start, stopping flow, incomplete emptying, and reduced stream [71]. Ruffo et al [62] reported a large study on 436 laparoscopic colon or rectal resections, in which careful nerve-sparing surgery was performed; nevertheless, 19.9% of patients suffered postoperative retention with a need for self-catheterization that persisted in 9.5% of patients after 1 month.

Finally, dysfunctional digestive symptoms are rarely studied; however, they should be a major concern in young and otherwise healthy women. Functional problems are not infrequent, being reported in up to 55% of cases and, although they may improve with time, tend to be permanent in a large percentage of patients. Functional sequelae may be related to "anterior rectal resection syndrome" or to autonomic nerve damage, and include severe constipation, tenesmus, and increase of daily stool [69]. Thomassin et al [33] reported de novo incidence of constipation and diarrhea in 55% of patients after surgery. Some symptoms are strongly dependent on the level of the anastomosis and, as in rectal cancer surgery, a better outcome is achieved when a colon pouch or a side-to-end anastomosis is performed [70].

3.2.5 Urinary Tract Endometriosis

3.2.5.1 Bladder Endometriosis

In cases of bladder endometriosis, the success of surgery, with long-lasting recovery from symptoms, typically correlates with how radical the exeresis is [72–77].

However, despite an adequate surgical exeresis, bladder endometriosis frequently recurs, at an estimated rate of 30%. Recurrences were documented to be inversely related to the patient's age.

Surgical management is generally recommended in women of fertile age who wish to become pregnant, since it is effective and ensures long-term relief in almost all cases [8, 24, 28]. Surgical exeresis of the lesions can be achieved using different procedures.

3.2.5.1.1 Transurethral Resection

Transurethral resection (TUR) might include both the bladder lesion and a 0.5–1-cm-deep portion of the adjacent myometrium, in order to reduce the percentage recurrence [74]. However, it should also be remembered that extensive TUR may induce a bladder perforation, thereby increasing the chance of recurrence itself, as reported by most authors [72, 78–82].

TUR should be considered in fertile patients due to its limited invasiveness. In order to achieve both radical exeresis and a low percentage of recurrence, it should be performed by skilled urologists.

3.2.5.1.2 Partial Cystectomy

Partial cystectomy (PC) is nowadays considered to be the treatment of choice for bladder endometriosis because it allows removal of the entire vesical lesion and prevents recurrence [83].

Nevertheless, PC is generally associated with precise criteria, which are: normal bladder function, normal bladder capacity, first diagnosis of bladder lesion, monofocality, and free margins in 1–2 cm. PC can be performed by either laparoscopy or laparotomy. The latter method is preferable, particularly in cases where the nodular lesion is located at the vesical base, as this location is frequently associated with severe and diffuse pelvic endometriosis.

Fedele et al [74] have reported a statistically significant reduction of recurrences when the resection included both the vesical lesion and a 0.5–1-cm-deep portion of the adjacent myometrium. Moreover, these authors suggested the laparotomic approach since this would permit better investigation of the ureters' integrity and performance of an accurate manual exploration of the detrusor and the involved myometrium.

As for bowel endometriosis, the laparoscopic approach is considered safe and effective, in skilled hands, although this approach also has to respect precise indications: the bladder lesion should be located far from bladder neck, ureteral meata, and trigone, and a precise preoperative definition of the lesion has to be obtained.

The technique, first described by Chapron and Dubuisson [84], and Nezhat et al [85], includes dissection of the vesico-uterine space in order to mobilize the nodule and dissect the bladder with excision of the whole nodule together with some healthy tissue. The bladder suture is generally performed by means of a single layer. Both groups advise a cystoscopy at the end of the procedure in order to ensure watertight closure and to check the integrity of the ureteral orifices. The outcomes were excellent in both series, with pain relief reported in 95% to 100% of patients [84, 85].

Patients who undergo a laparoscopic approach experience a shorter hospitalization time, a smaller incision, less adhesion formation, and faster recovery when compared to patients treated by open surgery. In addition, according to the literature, the laparoscopic approach improves the magnification of the operating field and will thus allow a more complete excision of the lesions [80, 84–87] (Figs. 3.9 and 3.10).

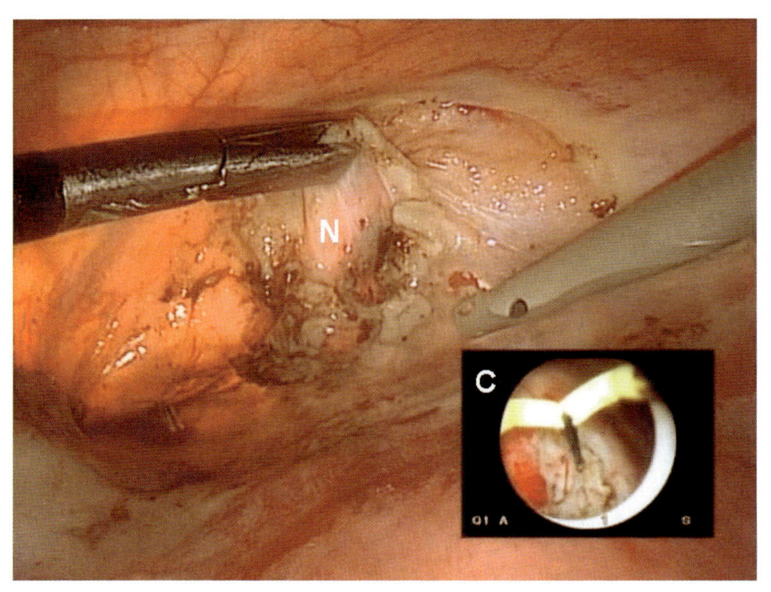

Fig. 3.9 Laparoscopic excision of bladder endometriosis. The nodule (*N*) deeply invades the bladder wall. A cystoscopy is simultaneously performed and is shown in the box (*C*)

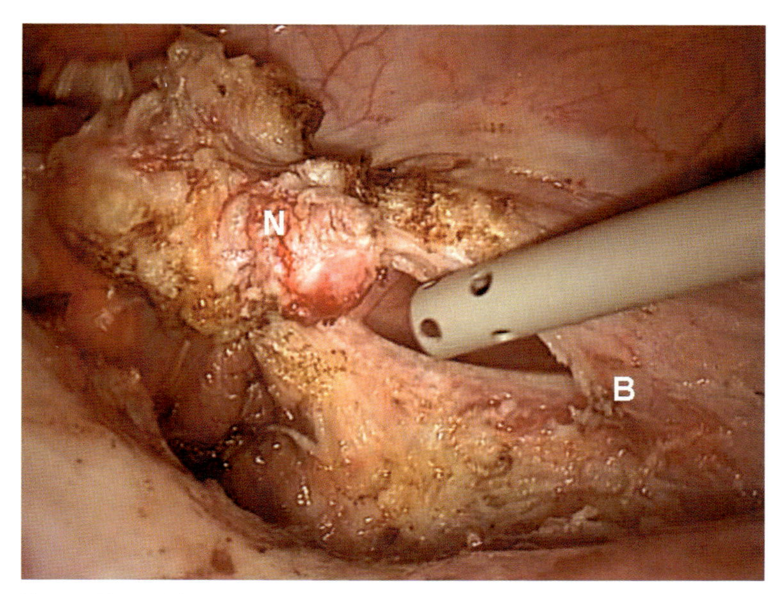

Fig. 3.10 The nodule (*N*) is being resected with opening of the bladder (*B*)

However, data concerning the laparoscopic treatment are only preliminary, due to the reduced series of patients and the difficult learning curve. Large multicenter studies are required before drawing definite conclusions [78, 88] and the long-term outcome needs to be evaluated [8, 24, 28, 89].

3.2.5.1.3
Combined Transurethral Partial Cystectomy and Laparoscopic Reconstruction of the Bladder

Combined transurethral partial cystectomy and laparoscopic reconstruction of the bladder for management of bladder endometriosis and coexisting abdominal endometriosis conform to the trend for minimally invasive surgery and might be considered as an alternative in experienced hands [90]. Sener et al have reported a similar case where surgery was performed with the aid of the da Vinci robot (Intuitive Surgical, Sunnyvale, CA, USA) [91]. Compared with standard laparoscopy, robot-assisted laparoscopy has the advantage of an improved level of freedom of instrumentation that might allow for an improved suturing technique. However, the longer set-up time and greater expense limits its use to only a few countries [91].

The association of hormonal therapy (HT) and surgical therapy (ST) might lead to a timely improvement of the symptoms, but the percentage of recurrence still remains high at about 35% [79, 92].

3.2.5.2 Ureteral Endometriosis

The main indications for surgical treatment of ureteral endometriosis (UE) are the presence of symptoms and/or hydro-ureteronephrosis [65, 93].

Historically, open surgery has been the preferred treatment in cases of extensive disease [94]. The success of surgery has been correlated with how radical the exeresis is; there is also a high risk of recurrence, estimated at 30%. This may in fact correspond to actual persistence of endometriotic lesions that were left in place as the result of an incomplete initial surgical removal [8, 24, 28].

Nowadays, laparoscopic interventions such as ureterolysis, ureterostomy, and ureteral reimplantation for ureteral stricture disease secondary to endometriosis can be performed, embracing the same principles of traditional urologic surgery, with magnified view, superior exposure, and greater ability to identify the disease in the pelvis and retroperitoneal space, as well as in the lower urinary tract [94–100].

Finally, current controversies in the treatment of UE concern when segmental resection and anastomosis, ureterolysis, or ureterocystoneostomy are best indicated, as well as whether minimal-access procedures are equally effective as the traditional open techniques [97, 98]. Generally, the choice of surgical treatment may change according to the diagnosis of intrinsic or extrinsic UE (Fig. 3.11).

Preoperative planning must be rigorous, and complete surgical excision of UE should be ensured by a team of experts who are familiar with endometriosis [101].

Moreover, the endometriosis itself increases the risk of ureteral trauma, which mostly occurs during surgery, in about 0.2–2% of cases [95, 102, 103]. As more complex procedures are increasingly performed by laparoscopy, the potential for operative injury to the ureter will inevitably increase [104]. About 70% of ureteral injuries are diagnosed postoperatively, and in more than two-thirds of cases, a laparotomy represents the favorite route for repair [102–107].

This underlines the necessity for appropriate tools to prevent and/or identify preoperatively any potential lesion.

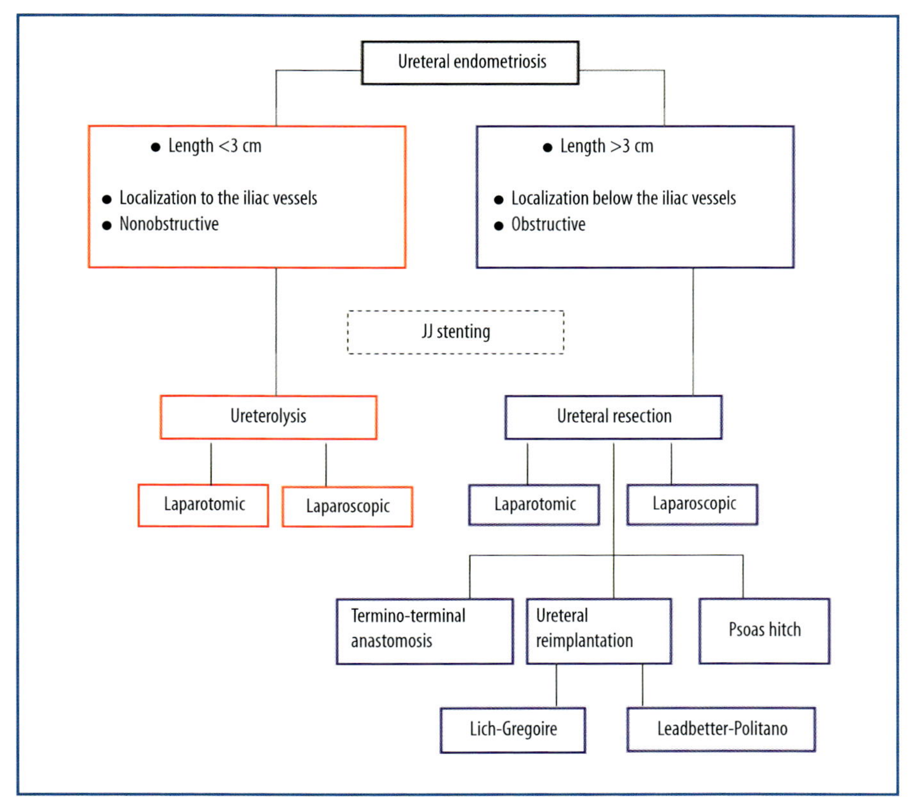

Fig. 3.11 Algorithm for surgical treatment of ureteral endometriosis

3.2.5.2.1
Extrinsic Ureteral Endometriosis

Elective ureterolysis should be indicated only when there is an extrinsic lesion that is smaller than 3 cm and/or nonobstructive ureteral involvement [72, 78, 97].

Preoperative or intraoperative use of a JJ stent is still controversial, with both a laparotomic and laparoscopic approach. Preoperative positioning before the procedure can guide the ureterolysis, especially in women with posterior nodules, and in the case of partial cystectomy when ureteral meata are adjacent to the lesion, it allows a more rapid identification of the ureter and can prevent ureteral lesions. On the other hand, the JJ, besides adding costs, increases the rigidity of the ureter thus making ureterolysis more difficult [104]. The JJ stent may also be positioned after ureterolysis, mainly to treat iatrogenic lesions created during surgery [108].

Ureterolysis is contraindicated in the case of intrinsic endometriosis due to both a high percentage of recurrence and ureteral stenosis.

3.2.5.2.2
Intrinsic Ureteral Endometriosis

Indications for ureteral resection include an intrinsic ureteral lesion and/or lesions that are longer than 3 cm, and a lesion site below the level of the iliac vessels [95, 109]. Traditionally, this type of surgery is performed by laparotomy, which is associated with some postoperative morbidity. Here too, the less invasive laparoscopic route may be considered [83].

The ureteral resection requires three techniques of ureteral reconstruction:

- ureteral termino-terminal anastomosis;
- ureteral reimplant with a antireflux technique (according to Lich–Gregoire or Leadbetter–Politano);
- the psoas hitch technique [101, 110–113].

A JJ stent may be a useful device as a permanent landmark for the surgeon during his resection/dissection, simplifying all the stages of re-anastomosis or reimplantation [108].

Despite all the ureteral surgical techniques, the percentage of deteriorated renal function still remains significant (40%). In these cases, nephrectomy may become necessary, also because the lesion sometimes mimics an urothelial carcinoma [114, 115].

Furthermore, it is advisable to perform an immunoistochemical examination for ER (estrogen receptors), PR (progesteron receptors), CK 7, CA 125, and CD 10 because of a high percentage of evolution into endometrioid carcinoma [115].

3.2.5.3
Kidney Endometriosis

Because DIE is generally characterized by high local aggressiveness and risk of recurrence, it requires surgical removal of the kidney masses (with either a laparotomic or laparoscopic approach), and eventually hormonal treatments, according to patient's age, symptoms, degree of obstruction, and the desire to preserve reproductive function [116–118].

Close follow-up is recommended, especially during the first 5 years after the intervention, with collaboration between the urologist and gynecologist.

3.2.5.4
Urethral Endometriosis

Only seven cases of urethral endometriosis have been reported in the literature; 4/7 patients have been previously diagnosed and treated for DIE, with both hormonal and surgical therapy [119–123].

The clinical presentation is like a cystic disease in which the vagina and urethra are involved. The treatment depends on the woman's age (relating to the desire for pregnancy), the extent of the disease, the alteration of the menstrual cycle, the sexual impact, and the presence of another pelvic disease [72, 119, 124]. The treatment options vary from watchful waiting (in nonsymptomatic patients) to a hormonal or surgical treatment, as in the other forms of urinary tract endometriosis. Nevertheless, when the size of urethral endometrioma is more than 2 cm, the elective treatment remains surgical excision [119, 121, 122, 124].

3.2.6
Repetitive Conservative Surgery

Surprisingly, only a few studies have addressed the efficacy of repeated conservative surgery for recurrent endometriosis, and no data are available specifically on reoperation for rectovaginal endometriosis. With the limited information available, symptomatic pain relapse has been reported in between 20% and 40% of women after repeated laparotomy [125]. The 24-month cumulative probability of dysmenorrhea and noncyclic pelvic pain after reintervention was estimated by Busacca et al to be 34% and 43% of patients, with no difference in patients operated on by laparoscopy or laparotomy, although the number of patients requiring a third intervention was higher in the latter group [126].

The cumulative probability of further surgery is between 15% and 20%. Operations for recurrence are usually more difficult and risky.

3

3.2.7 Definitive Surgery

For women with repeated failure of conservative surgical treatment, the definitive therapy consists of total hysterectomy and bilateral salphingo-oophorectomy, with removal of all endometriotic tissue, in particular lesions involving the pouch of Douglas [127].

Symptomatic recurrence has, in fact, been observed even after nonconservative surgery. Fedele et al [128] studied 38 women who underwent definitive surgery with a minimum follow-up of 24 months; only the group of patients in whom radical surgery was associated with removal of all endometriotic lesions showed no recurrence.

After radical surgery, hormone replacement therapy is usually administered, to prevent postmenopausal symptoms and problems. This therapy could possibly reactivate endometriotic lesions that have not been removed during hysterosalphingectomy [128].

Aknowledgments This chapter has been written in collaboration with R. Colombo and C. Macagnano (Department of Urology, San Raffaele Scientific Institute, Milan, Italy).

References

1. Mechsner S, Bartley J, Loddenkemper C et al. Oxytocin receptor expression in smooth muscle cells of peritoneal endometriotic lesions and ovarian endometriotic cysts. Fertil Steril 2005;83(S1):1220–1231
2. Bulun SE. Endometriosis. N Engl J Med 2009;360:268–279
3. Ferrero S, Gillott DJ, Remorgida V et al. Proteomics technologies in endometriosis. Expert Rev Proteomics 2008;5:705–714
4. Ebert AD, Jakisch D, Müller MD et al. Endometriosezentren verschiedener Stufen zur Verbesserung der medizinischen Versorgungsqualität, der Forschung sowie der ärztlichen Fort- und Weiterbildung. J Gynäkol Endokrinol 2008;18:62–68
5. Garry R. The effectiveness of laparoscopic excision of endometriosis. Curr Opin Obstet Gynecol 2004;16:299–303
6. Davis CJ, McMillan L. Pain in endometriosis: effectiveness of medical and surgical management. Curr Opin Obstet Gynecol 2003;15:507–512
7. Jacobson TZ, Barlow DH, Garry R, Koninckx P. Laparoscopic surgery for pelvic pain associated with endometriosis. Cochrane Database Syst Rev 2009;4:CD001300
8. Fedele L, Bianchi S, Zanconato G et al. Is rectovaginal endometriosis a progressive disease? Am J Obstet Gynecol 2004;191:1539–1542
9. Chapron C, Dubuisson JB, Chopin N et al. Deeply infiltrating endometriosis: management and proposal for a "surgical classification". Gynecol Obstet Fertil 2003;31:197–206
10. De Nardi P, Osman N, Ferrari S et al. Laparoscopic treatment of deep pelvic endometriosis with rectal involvement. Dis Colon Rectum 2009;52:419–424

11. Chapron C, Dubuisson J-B. Management of deep endometriosis. Ann NY Acad Sci 2001;943:276–280
12. Chapron C, Fauconnier A, Vieira M et al. Anatomical distribution of deeply infiltrating endometriosis: surgical implications and proposition for a classification. Hum Reprod 2003;18:157–161
13. Brouwer R, Woods RJ. Rectal endometriosis: results of radical excision and review of published work. ANZ J Surg 2007;77:562–571
14. Jerby BL, Kessler H, Falcone T, Milsom JW. Laparoscopic management of colorectal endometriosis. Surg Endosc 1999;13:1125–1128
15. Davis CJ, McMillan L. Pain in endometriosis: effectiveness of medical and surgical Management. Curr Opin Obstet Gynecol 2003;15:507–512
16. Doyle JB. Paracervical uterine denervation by transection of the cervical plexus for the relief of dysmenorrhea. Am J Obstet Gynecol 1955;70:1–16
17. Proctor ML, Latthe PM, Farquhar CM et al. Surgical interruption of pelvic nerve pathways for primary and secondary dysmenorrhoea. Cochrane Database Syst Rev 2005;(4):CD001896
18. Johnson NP, Farquhar CM, Crossley S et al. A double-blind randomised controlled trial of laparoscopic uterine nerve ablation for women with chronic pelvic pain. Int J Obstet Gynecol 2004;111:950–959
19. Sutton C, Pooley AS, Jones KD et al. A prospective, randomised, double blind controlled trial of laparoscopic uterine nerve ablation in the treatment of pelvic pain associated with endometriosis. Gynecol Endosc 2001;10:217–222
20. Lichten EM, Bormbard J. Surgical treatment of primary dysmenorrhea with laparoscopic uterine nerve ablation. J Reprod Med 1987;32:37–41
21. Candiani GB, Fedele L, Vercellini P et al. Presacral neurectomy for the treatment of pelvic pain associated with endometriosis: a controlled study. Am J Obstet Gynecol 1992;167:100–103
22. Kwok A, Lam A, Ford R. Laparoscopic presacral neurectomy: a review. Obstet Gynecol Surv 2001;56:99–104
23. Soysal ME, Soysal S, Gurses E, Ozer S. Laparoscopic presacral neurolysis for endometriosis-related pelvic pain. Hum Reprod 2003;18:588–592
24. Redwine DB, Wright JT. Laparoscopic treatment of complete obliteration of the cul-de-sac associated with endometriosis: long-term follow-up of en bloc resection. Fertil Steril 2001;76:358–365
25. Abrão MS, Neme RM, Averbach M. Endometriose de septo reto-vaginal: doença de diagnóstico e tratamento específicos. Arq Gastroenterol 2003;40:192–197
26. Angioni S, Peiretti M, Zirone M et al. Laparoscopic excision of posterior vaginal fornix in the treatment of patients with deep endometriosis without rectum involvement: surgical treatment and long-term follow-up. Hum Reprod 2006;21:1629–1634
27. Chapron C, Jacob S, Dubuisson J-B et al. Laparoscopically assisted vaginal management of deep endometriosis infiltrating the rectovaginal septum. Acta Obstet Gynecol Scand 2001;80:349–354
28. Fedele L, Bianchi S, Zanconato G et al. Long-term follow-up after conservative surgery for rectovaginal endometriosis. Am J Obstet Gynecol 2004;190:1020–1024
29. Campagnacci R, Perretta S, Guerrieri M et al. Laparoscopic colorectal resection for endometriosis. Surg Endosc 2005;19:662–664
30. Bailey HR, Ott MT, Hartendorp P. Aggressive surgical management for advanced colorectal endometriosis. Dis Colon Rectum 1994;37:747–752
31. Urbach DR, Reedijk M, Richard CS et al. Bowel resection for intestinal endometriosis. Dis Colon Rectum 1998;41:1158–1164
32. Mourthé de Alvim Andrade M, Batista Pimenta M, de Freitas Belezia B, Duarte T. Rectal obstruction due to endometriosis. Tech Coloproctol 2008;12:57–59

3

33. Thomassin I, Bazot M, Detchev R et al. Symptoms before and after surgical removal of colorectal endometriosis that are assessed by magnetic resonance imaging and rectal endoscopic sonography. Am J Obstet Gynecol 2004;190:1264–1271
34. Darai E, Thomassin I, Barranger E et al. Feasibility and clinical outcome of laparoscopic colorectal resection for endometriosis. Am J Obstet Gynecol 2005;192:394–400
35. Remorgida V, Ferrero S, Fulcheri E et al. Bowel endometriosis: presentation, diagnosis, and treatment. Obstetric Gynecol Surv 2007;62:461–470
36. Healey M, Ang WC, Cheng C. Surgical treatment of endometriosis: a prospective randomized double-blinded trial comparing excision and ablation. Fertil Steril 2010;March 30 [epub ahead of print]
37. Donnez J, Squifflet J. Complications, pregnancy and recurrence in a prospective series of 500 patients operated on by the shaving technique for deep rectovaginal endometriotic nodules. Human Reproduction, 2010;25(8):1949–1958
38. Nezhat C, Nezhat F, Pennington E et al. Laparoscopic disk excision and primary repair of the anterior rectal wall for the treatment of full-thickness endometriosis. Surg Endosc 1994;8:682–685
39. Gordon SJ, Maher PJ, Woods R. Use of the CEEA stapler to avoid ultra-low segmental resection of a full-thickness rectal endometriotic nodule. J Am Assoc Gynecol Laparosc 2001;8:312–316
40. Woods RJ, Heriot AG, Chen FC. Anterior rectal wall excision for endometriosis using the circular stapler. ANZ J Surg 2003;73:647–648
41. Reich H. Laparoscopic hysterectomy for advanced endometriosis. In: Jain N (ed) Atlas of endoscopic surgery in infertility and gynecology. McGraw-Hill, New York (NY), 2004, pp 298–320
42. Remorgida V, Ragni N, Ferrero S et al. The involvement of the interstitial Cajal cells and the enteric nervous system in bowel endometriosis. Hum Reprod 2005;20:264–271
43. Remorgida V, Ragni N, Ferrero S et al. How complete is full thickness disc resection of bowel endometriotic lesions? A prospective surgical and histological study. Hum Reprod 2005;20:2317–2320
44. Anaf V, El Nakadi I, Simon P et al. Preferential infiltration of large bowel endometriosis along the nerves of the colon. Hum Reprod 2004;19:996–1002
45. Abrão MS, Podgaec S, Dias JA Jr et al. Endometriosis lesions that compromise the rectum deeper than the inner muscularis layer have more than 40% of the circumference of the rectum affected by the disease. J Minim Invasive Gynecol 2008;15:280–285
46. Kavallaris A, Koèhler C, Kuèhne-Heid R, Schneider A. Histopathological extent of rectal invasion by rectovaginal endometriosis. Hum Reprod 2003;18:1323–1327
47. Roman H. Guidelines for the management of painful endometriosis. J Gynecol Obstet Biol Reprod 2007;33:141–150
48. Roman H, Opris I, Resch B et al. Histopathologic features of endometriotic rectal nodules and the implications for management by rectal nodule excision. Fertil Steril 2009;92:1250–1252
49. Busacca M, Somigliana E, Bianchi S et al. Post-operative GnRH analogue treatment after conservative surgery for symptomatic endometriosis stage III–IV: a randomized controlled trial. Hum Reprod 2001;16:2399–2402
50. Nezhat F, Nezhat C, Pennington E. Laparoscopic proctectomy for infiltrating endometriosis of the rectum. Fertil Steril 1992;57:1129–1132
51. Redwine DB, Koning M, Sharpe DR. Laparoscopically assisted transvaginal segmental resection of the rectosigmoid colon for endometriosis. Fertil Steril 1996;65:193–197
52. Fleisch MC, Xafis D, De Bruyne F et al. Radical resection of invasive endometriosis with bowel or bladder involvement – long-term results. Eur J Obstet Gynecol Reprod Biol 2005; 123:224–229
53. Abbott A, Hawe J, Clayton RD, Garry R. The effects and effectiveness of laparoscopic exci-

sion of endometriosis: a prospective study with 2 ± 5 year follow-up. J Hum Reprod 2003;18:1922–1927
54. Darai E, Ackerman G, Bazot M et al. Laparoscopic segmental colorectal resection for endometriosis: limits and complications. Surg Endosc 2007;21:1572–1577
55. Seracchioli R, Poggioli G, Pierangeli F et al. Surgical outcome and long-term follow up after laparoscopic rectosigmoid resection in women with deep infiltrating endometriosis. BJOG 2007;114:889–895
56. Busacca M, Chiaffarino F, Candiani M et al. Determinants of long-term clinically detected recurrence rates of deep, ovarian, and pelvic endometriosis. Am J Obstet Gynecol 2006;195:426–432
57. Redwine DB, Sharpe DR. Laparoscopic segmental resection of the sigmoid colon for endometriosis. J Laparoendosc Surg 1991;1:217–220
58. Duepree HJ, Senagore AJ, Delaney CP et al. Laparoscopic resection of deep pelvic endometriosis with rectosigmoid involvement. J Am Coll Surg 2002;195:254–258
59. Marpeau O, Thomassin I, Barranger E et al. Résection coelioscopique du colon-rectum pour endométriose: résultats preliminaires. J Gynecol Obstet Biol Reprod 2004;33:600–606
60. Dubernard G, Piketty M, Rouzier R et al. Quality of life after laparoscopic colorectal resection for endometriosis. Hum Reprod 2006;21:1243–1247
61. Mereu L, Ruffo G, Landi S et al. Laparoscopic treatment of deep endometriosis with segmental colorectal resection: short-term morbidity. J Minim Invasive Gynecol 2007;14:463–469
62. Ruffo G, Scopelliti F, Scioscia M et al. Laparoscopic colorectal resection for deep infiltrating endometriosis: analysis of 436 cases. Surg Endosc 2010;24:63–67
63. Fayez J, Collazo LM. Comparison between laparotomy and operative laparoscopy in the treatment of moderate and severe endometriosis. Int J Fertil 1990;35:272–279
64. Crosignani PG, Vercellini P, Biffignandi F et al. Laparoscopy versus laparotomy in conservative surgical treatment for severe endometriosis. Fertil Steril 1996;66:706–711
65. Darai E, Dubernard G, Coutant C et al. Randomized trial of laparoscopically assisted versus open colorectal resection for endometriosis morbidity, symptoms, quality of life, and fertility. Ann Surg 2010;251:1018–1023
66. Ford J, English J, Miles WA, Giannopoulos T. Pain, quality of life and complications following the radical resection of rectovaginal endometriosis. Int J Gynaecol Obstet 2004;111:353–356
67. Benbara A, Fortin B, Martin L et al. Résection rectosigmoidienne pour endométriose profonde: resultats chirurgicaux et fonctionnels. [Surgical and functional results of colorectal resection for severe endometriosis.] Gynecol Obstet Fertil 2008;36:1191–1201
68. Golfier F, Sabra M. Surgical management of endometriosis. J Gynecol Obstet Biolog Reprod 2007;36:162–172
69. Roman H, Loise C, Resch B et al. Delayed functional outcomes associated with surgical management of deep rectovaginal endometriosis with rectal involvement: giving patients an informed choice. Hum Reprod 2010;25(4):890–899
70. Ret Dávalos ML, De Cicco C, D'Hoore A et al. Outcome after rectum or sigmoid resection: a review for gynecologists. J Min Inv Gynecol 2007;14:33–38
71. Dubernard G, Rouzier R, David-Montefiore E et al. Urinary complications after surgery for posterior deep infiltrating endometriosis are related to the extent of dissection and to uterosacral ligaments resection. J Minim Invasive Gynecol 2008;15:235–240
72. Comiter CV. Endometriosis of the urinary tract. Urol Clin North Am 2002;29:625–635
73. Donnez J, Van Langendonckt A, Casanas-Roux F et al. Current thinking on the pathogenesis of endometriosis. Gynecol Obstet Invest 2002;54(S1):52–58
74. Fedele L, Bianchi S, Zanconato G et al. Long-term follow-up after conservative surgery for bladder endometriosis. Fertil Steril 2005;83:1729–1733
75. Garry R. Endometrial ablation and resection: validation of a new surgical concept. Br J Obstet Gynaecol 1997;104:1329–1331

76. Chopin N, Vieira M, Borghese B et al. Operative management of deeply infiltrating endometriosis: results on pelvic pain symptoms according to a surgical classification. J Minim Invasive Gynecol 2005;12:106–112
77. Vignali M, Bianchi S, Candiani M et al. Surgical treatment of deep endometriosis and risk of recurrence. J Minim Invasive Gynecol 2005;12:508–513
78. Antonelli A, Simeone C, Canossi E et al. Surgical approach to urinary endometriosis: experience on 28 cases. Arch Ital Urol Androl 2006;78:35–38
79. Gustilo-Ashby AM, Paraiso MF. Treatment of urinary tract endometriosis. J Minim Invasive Gynecol 2006;13:559–565
80. Granese R, Candiani M, Perino A et al. Bladder endometriosis: laparoscopic treatment and follow-up. Eur J Obstet Gynecol Reprod Biol 2008;140:114–117
81. Vercellini P, Meschia M, De Giorgi O et al. Bladder detrusor endometriosis: clinical and pathogenetic implications. J Urol 1996;155:84–86
82. Dubuisson JB, Chapron C. Classification of endometriosis. The need for modification. Hum Reprod 1994;9:2214–2216
83. Seracchioli R, Mabrouk M, Montanari G et al. Conservative laparoscopic management of urinary tract endometriosis (UTE): surgical outcome and long-term follow-up. Fertil Steril 2010;94:856–861
84. Chapron C, Dubuisson JB. Laparoscopic management of bladder endometriosis. Acta Obstet Gynecol Scand 1999;78:887–890
85. Nezhat C, Nezhat F, Nezhat CH et al. Urinary tract endometriosis treated by laparoscopy. Fertil Steril 1996;66:920–924
86. Nezhat CH, Malik S, Osias J et al. Laparoscopic management of 15 patients with infiltrating endometriosis of the bladder and a case of primary intravesical endometrioid adenosarcoma. Fertil Steril 2002;78:872–875
87. Chapron C, Dubuisson JB, Jacob S et al. Laparoscopy and bladder endometriosis. Gynecol Obstet Fertil 2000;28:232–237
88. Donnez J, Spada F, Squifflet J, Nisolle M. Bladder endometriosis must be considered as bladder adenomyosis. Fertil Steril 2000;74:1175–1181
89. Chapron C, Bourret A, Chopin N et al. Surgery for bladder endometriosis: long-term results and concomitant management of associated posterior deep lesions. Hum Reprod 2010;25:884–889
90. Pang ST, Chao A, Wang CJ et al. Transurethral partial cystectomy and laparoscopic reconstruction for the management of bladder endometriosis. Fertil Steril 2008;90:2014
91. Sener A, Chew BH, Duvdevani M et al. Combined transurethral and laparoscopic partial cystectomy and robot-assisted bladder repair for the treatment of bladder endometrioma. J Minim Invasive Gynecol 2006;13:245–248
92. Pastor-Navarro H, Giménez-Bachs JM, Donate-Moreno MJ et al. Update on the diagnosis and treatment of bladder endometriosis. Int Urogynecol J Pelvic Floor Dysfunct 2007;18:949–954
93. Collinet P, Marcelli F, Villers A et al. Management of endometriosis of the urinary tract. Gynecol Obstet Fertil 2006;34:347–352
94. Douglas C, Rotimi O. Extragenital endometriosis – a clinicopathological review of a Glasgow hospital experience with case illustrations. J Obstet Gynaecol 2004;24:804–808
95. Yohannes P. Ureteral endometriosis. J Urol 2003;170:20–25
96. Kinkel K, Frei KA, Balleyguier C, Chapron C. Diagnosis of endometriosis with imaging: a review. Eur Radiol 2006;16:285–298
97. Frenna V, Santos L, Ohana E et al. Laparoscopic management of ureteral endometriosis: our experience. J Minim Invasive Gynecol 2007;14:169–171
98. Nezhat C, Silfen S, Nezhat F, Martin D. Surgery for endometriosis. Curr Opin Obstet Gynecol 1991;3:385–393

99. Chung H, Jeong BC, Kim HH. Laparoscopic ureteroneocystostomy with vesicopsoas hitch: nonrefluxing ureteral reimplantation using cystoscopy-assisted submucosal tunneling. J Endourol 2006;20:632–638
100. Ghezzi F, Cromi A, Bergamini V et al. Outcome of laparoscopic ureterolysis for ureteral endometriosis. Fertil Steril 2006;86:418–422
101. Mereu L, Gagliardi ML, Clarizia R et al. Laparoscopic management of ureteral endometriosis in case of moderate-severe hydroureteronephrosis. Fertil Steril 2010;93:46–51
102. Grainger DA, Soderstrom RM, Schiff SF et al. Ureteral injuries at laparoscopy: insights into diagnosis, management and prevention. Obstet Gynecol 1990;76:889–890
103. Rafique M, Arif MH. Management of iatrogenic ureteric injuries associated with gynaecological surgery. Int Urol Nephrol 2002;34:31–35
104. Assimos DG, Patterson LC, Taylor CL. Changing incidence and etiology of iatrogenic ureteral injuries. J Urol 1994;152:2240–2246
105. Ostrzenski A, Radolinski B, Ostrzenska KM. A review of laparoscopic ureteral injury in pelvic surgery. Obstet Gynecol Surv 2003;58:794–799
106. Giannakopoulos X, Lolis D, Grammeniatis E, Kotoulas K. Iatrogenic injuries to the distal ureter during gynaecologic interventions. J Urol 1995;101:69
107. Saidi MH, Sadler RK, Vancaillie TG et al. Diagnosis and management of serious urinary complications after major operative laparoscopy. Obstet Gynecol 1996;87:272–276
108. Weingertner AS, Rodriguez B, Ziane A et al. The use of JJ stent in the management of deep endometriosis lesion, affecting or potentially affecting the ureter: a review of our practice. BJOG 2008;115:1159–1164
109. Marcelli F, Collinet P, Vinatier D et al. Ureteric and bladder involvement of deep pelvic endometriosis. Value of multidisciplinary surgical management. Prog Urol 2006;16:588–593
110. Seracchioli R, Mannini D, Colombo FM et al. Cystoscopy-assisted laparoscopic resection of extramucosal bladder endometriosis. J Endourol 2002;16:663–666
111. Carmignani L, Ronchetti A, Amicarelli F et al. Bladder psoas hitch in hydronephrosis due to pelvic endometriosis: outcome of urodynamic parameters. Fertil Steril 2009;92:35–40
112. Bondavalli C, Dall'Oglio B, Schiavon L et al. Pathology of the gynecologic ureter: our experience. Arch Ital Urol Androl 2002;74:25–26
113. Chapron C, Pietin-Vialle C, Borghese B et al. Associated ovarian endometrioma is a marker for greater severity of deeply infiltrating endometriosis. Fertil Steril 2009;92:453–457
114. Klein RS, Cattolica EV. Ureteral endometriosis. Urology 1979;13:477–482
115. Al-Khawaja M, Tan PH, MacLennan GT et al. Ureteral endometriosis: clinicopathological and immunohistochemical study of 7 cases. Hum Pathol 2008;39:954–959
116. Olive DL, Pritts EA. Treatment of endometriosis. N Engl J Med 2001;345:266–275
117. Nezhat C, Nezhat F, Nezhat CH et al. Urinary tract endometriosis treated by laparoscopy. Fertil Steril 1996;66:920–924
118. Dirim A, Celikkaya S, Aygun C, Caylak B. Renal endometriosis presenting with a giant subcapsular hematoma: case report. Fertil Steril 2009;92:391
119. Cabral Ribeiro J, Pérez García D, Martins Silva C, Ribeiro Santos A. Suburethral endometrioma. Actas Urol Esp 2007;31:153–156
120. Pałczyński B, Blok K, Blok R et al. Urethral obstruction caused by endometriosis. Ginekol Pol 2002;73:853–855
121. Chowdhry AA, Miller FH, Hammer RA. Endometriosis presenting as a urethral diverticulum: a case report. J Reprod Med 2004;49:321–323
122. Wu YC, Liang CC, Soong YK. Suburethral endometrioma. A case report. J Reprod Med 2003;48:204–205
123. Arzoz Fabregas M, Ibarz Servio L, Areal Calama J, Saladie Roig JM. Divertículos de uretra femenina. Arch Esp Urol 2004,57:381–388

124. Frackiewicz EJ. Endometriosis: an overview of the disease and its treatment. J Am Pharm Assoc 2000;40:645–657
125. Vercellini P, Barbara G, Abbiati A et al. Repetitive surgery for recurrent symptomatic endometriosis: what to do? Eur J Obstet Gynecol Reprod Biol 2009;146:15–21
126. Busacca, L Fedele, S Bianchi et al. Surgical treatment of recurrent endometriosis: laparotomy versus laparoscopy. Hum Reprod 1998;13:2271–2274
127. Berlanda N, Vercellini P, Fedele L. The outcomes of repeat surgery for recurrent symptomatic endometriosis. Curr Opin Obstet Gynecol 2010;22:320–325
128. Fedele L, Bianchi S, Zanconato G et al. Tailoring radicality in demolitive surgery for deeply infiltrating endometriosis. Am J Obstet Gynecol 2005;193:114–117

The Experience of Living with Endometriosis

4

E. Denny

Abstract The experience of endometriosis can impact on every aspect of a woman's life and of those around her, although the range of experience is diverse. Using qualitative research undertaken with women with endometriosis, this chapter explores the experiences that are most frequently reported. It begins by considering the well-documented delay in diagnosis, and comments on the impact that receiving a diagnosis can have. It then moves on to explore the pain of endometriosis, and the way in which women describe this. A particular type of pain that is common in endometriosis is dyspareunia and this is discussed along with fertility, as both are important aspects of sexuality that may be disrupted by endometriosis. The impact of endometriosis on a woman's life is played out in her social relationships, her interactions with health professionals, and her experience of interventions and treatments. These issues are presented in remainder of the chapter. Through the words of women with endometriosis, the impact of the disease is brought into sharp relief.

Keywords Impact of endometriosis • Illness experience • Qualitative research • Pain • Fertility

E. Denny (✉)
Professor of Health Sociology, Faculty of Health, Birmingham City University, Birmingham, UK

Deep Pelvic Endometriosis. Paola De Nardi, Stefano Ferrari

4.1 Introduction

It is well known that endometriosis impacts on quality of life in a number of ways. Different women will endure a greater or lesser degree of symptomatology, which is not necessarily related to the extent or severity of disease. The experience may range from a minor irritation to a life totally overwhelmed by endometriosis. Even within one woman, the disease pattern may alter at different stages of her life. So a chapter on women's experience of endometriosis has first to acknowledge that there is great diversity in that experience, and uncertainty as to how it will manifest in the future. Nevertheless there has been a body of research over the past few years that has produced fairly consistent results on the impact of living with symptomatic endometriosis, and this research will be utilized here to capture the reality for those women whose lives are affected by it. Much of this research has been conducted using qualitative methodological approaches that give women a voice to tell their stories of life with endometriosis and the sense they make of it. These narratives have provided detailed and salient data that have increased the knowledge base of this disease beyond the clinical and scientific. Women's voices will provide the quotations that are included here, which are taken from research presented in full elsewhere [1–5].

4.2 Diagnosis of Endometriosis

4.2.1 Delay in Diagnosis

Delay in diagnosis has been a consistent finding in the literature [2, 6, 7], and Ballard et al have described this as either doctor delay or patient delay [7]. Patient delays frequently occur because women do not recognise their symptoms as "not normal" – sometimes because this all they have known since the menarche, and sometimes because they have an expectation of menstruation as painful. Women often say that they think they are unlucky to suffer from painful periods, or that it is all part of womanhood.

> "I always suffered from quite bad periods, painful periods, heavy bleeding for the first couple of days every cycle . . . It just became a way of life. It became the norm and I assumed that's just what happens." [5]

Relatives can also reinforce this thinking.

> "I discussed it with my mum and she said 'don't worry about that, I had painful periods and when you have your first child that will all go'." [2]

Doctor delays occur when women do seek medical help and are either referred to the wrong specialist or not taken seriously.

> "I went to the doctor's and he said 'Women do suffer with painful periods, it's one of those things'." [2]

> "I was seeing a female doctor and I remember thinking great, she will have some sympathy. She just told me all women have to put up with it." [5]

Women report doctors telling them that it is what all women go through, or that they are being weak and should put up with pain, so that women will either endure it or embark on the "medical merry go round" [6], trying to find a doctor who will take them seriously. This can sometimes take many years, adding to delays in diagnosis, and has been referred to as "doctor shopping" [8]. This pejorative term however belies the trauma for women of being dismissed time and again when seeking answers to the pain.

Normalization of pain is frequently directed at young women and adolescents who are told that they will grow out of it, or that the pain will stop when they have children (myths that are discussed below). Those women who have excessive pain from the onset of menarche seem most likely to have a negative experience, raising questions about how adolescents are stereotyped in the medical profession. Conversely, women whose symptoms began later in life are more able to argue effectively that there is a difference between present and previous experience.

4.2.2 Impact of a Diagnosis of Endometriosis

Diagnosis is integral to the theory and practice of modern western medicine, and for the patient it gives a name to something that has previously been unknown. For patients with endometriosis it confirms the reality of their pain, and this is particularly true when women have felt disbelieved or "fobbed off", which is a phrase used by many women. Women report feeling relieved to receive a diagnosis and say it is a vindication of their persistence in seeking medical help for their symptoms.

> "When I came round, I felt like saying, 'told you so'. I really felt quite smug for about 5 minutes until it hit me, I thought, 'no that's not the outcome I actually wanted'. For once, I wanted to be wrong but it's just annoying that they didn't really want to listen to me." [5]

Women have also been reported as finding symptoms easier to deal with once it is known they have a condition they can name [7], and as feeling they have credibility in their interactions with health professionals. A diagnostic label also helps women to have legitimacy among their peer group and work colleagues when they withdraw from normal activities, which will be discussed further below. For women with endometriosis, seeing their lesions on photographs and videos provides a visible image that adds to their sense of legitimacy, and helps them to make sense of their experience.

Following the relief and vindication however, women often feel anger that they have been disbelieved, and are left wondering about the implications of the delay.

> "When they gave me my endo diagnosis I was fuming that I hadn't been believed and that I hadn't been taken seriously . . . I was actually convinced by a doctor that I was psychosomatic and a bit of a hypochondriac." [2]

> "I do feel angry because if they'd realised it before and done something about it earlier, the situation perhaps could have been completely different. I think I suffered almost 9 years." [2]

4.2.3 Pain

From the discussion above it can be seen that both women themselves and health professionals have difficulty in differentiating "normal" from "abnormal" menstrual pain, the physiological from the pathological. However, pain is highly subjective and there is no objective measure by which women and their doctors can differentiate between "normal" and "abnormal" pain, and so it is important to women to be believed and treated as credible. The experience of endometriosis is compounded by pain being trivialized or normalized, and being taken seriously becomes of utmost importance. For some women, pain is not only associated with menstruation, but is constant, or is accompanied by deep dyspareunia (discussed below), dyschezia, or dysuria, and these pains may be more likely to be labeled as "not normal". The descriptions of pain that women give during interviews help to explain the impact that it has on their lives. Words such as "stabbing", "like a knife in both ovaries", and "grinding" are used to attempt to portray the chronic and debilitating nature of the pain. For some women this is cyclical, and in between they can carry on life as normal (albeit with the knowledge that the pain will return in a few weeks), but for some women pain is a constant in their lives, maybe waxing and waning, but never leaving them.

> "When it's at its worst is when the last thing that you remember before you fall asleep is that you're in pain, and before you are even aware you're awake you're aware you are in pain." [1]

> "The best way I can describe it is if you sort of imagine someone with nails sort of clawing inside your stomach, it's that intense and it almost comes in waves." [1]

Data from a small sample of women who kept diaries suggest that symptoms are mainly dealt with using over-the-counter medication, sometimes supplemented by prescription drugs that they will learn to take in combinations for the best effect [5].

Some women will try to accommodate the pain into their lives and not be dominated by it, while others find it overwhelming and cannot imagine a life without pain. One of the problems for women in attempting to have their pain taken seriously is that menstrual pain is generally seen as a low-status pain. It does not have the same impact in the imagination of lay or professional people as, for example, the pain of cancer [5]. Menstrual pain is widely experienced, and, like back pain, may be associated with malingering. In addition, endometriosis is not a disease that has a high profile, nor is it life threatening, so it is not of interest to many in the medical profession.

> "It's not a sexy disease. It's not life threatening, so there is very little interest." [5]

> "It's a hard illness because you don't die of it and therefore it is given a secondary importance." [5]

4.3 Sexuality

4.3.1 Dyspareunia

One of the most distressing manifestations of pain, which affects a woman's self-esteem and relationships, is dyspareunia on deep penetration. Sexual intimacy is a fundamental aspect of humanity, and the inability to engage in mutually satisfying sexual activity may have a profound effect on self-esteem and on relationships with partners [5]. The extent to which women with endometriosis experience this has been reported as between 60.6% and 86% [3]. This range of findings may be because women will not volunteer information on a highly personal subject [1]. Many women avoid sexual intercourse because of dyspareunia, or stop when it becomes too painful, and some experience pain for many hours following penetrative sex. Although women report that their quality of life is negatively affected by dyspareunia, the extent to which this occurs varies.

> "Obviously sex was painful and that would cause a problem because I wouldn't be able to have sex quite as much, it would be uncomfortable and painful for days afterwards. That put a strain on the relationship." [1]

> "I felt guilty and inadequate because I didn't want sex, and my only way of dealing with it has been to cut off and I've felt that I blame myself, and feel inadequate." [3]

Women feel guilty at avoiding sexual intercourse, and they also feel unfeminine, but younger women in less stable relationships have been shown to be more acutely affected, with women in established relationships being more philosophical and valuing other aspects of their relationship [3]. The relative importance of an active sex life compared with other aspects of the relationship is often lower in this group, but assumptions cannot be made based solely on age and length of relationship. Dyspareunia can place a lot of strain on a relationship, causing great tension, and with some ending in separation. Women do often report their partner as being supportive, but even this is qualified, and negative effects on the partner are also commented on.

> "He has been great, really excellent. There are times when there is friction because it does get to him, understandably." [3]

4.3.2 Fertility

Despite experiencing dyspareunia, some women will endure the pain, and this is usually because the desire for a pregnancy is paramount. Indeed for some women, the most important aspect of endometriosis is the actual or perceived effect on fertility.

"My GP was saying, 'Let [conception] happen naturally', and I was saying, 'It's impossible to try during my ovulation time. I am in agony, and I'm trying to have sex and it's just not happening'." [1]

This is particularly true for those women who are symptomless and only diagnosed during fertility investigations. The anxiety caused by the inability to conceive is compounded by a diagnosis of endometriosis, although endometriosis may be of secondary importance. Nulliparous women with symptomatic endometriosis who have no immediate desire to conceive are frequently concerned about their future fertility, and this is a real issue for women who are offered treatments that suppress their normal menstrual cycle.

"Obviously I am still concerned that should there be any remaining endometriosis, this may affect my fertility." [5]

4.4 Uncertainty

As with many chronic and long-term conditions, the trajectory of endometriosis is surrounded by uncertainty. Uncertainty around diagnosis has been discussed above, and women may be given incorrect diagnoses on the way to discovering that they have endometriosis. Irritable bowel syndrome (IBS) is one of the most common (mis)diagnoses that women receive [2], but being labeled as depressed is also common, or as anxious over not achieving a pregnancy.

"I went to the doctor . . . and he sent me up to the hospital to get a scan on my ovaries which showed clear. So then he decided it was IBS and I was back and forth from the doctor for weeks on different treatments which didn't make any difference at all." [2]

Some women are also led to believe that their symptoms are psychosomatic.

"It hasn't helped my self-image or confidence to be told for the best part of 14 years that I was imagining it or overreacting, I needed to see a psychiatrist."

However, having a diagnosis does not ensure a smooth patient journey. The significance of symptoms for a doctor is in guiding them to the correct diagnosis and for evaluation of treatment, whereas for the patient the effect on their quality of life and interference with social functioning might be paramount [5]. For example, the medical concern regarding pain is generally the site and level of pain, which is usually gauged by pain scores, but for a woman with endometriosis the duration and quality of pain are also of major importance in determining her ability to function and maintain social relationships. The randomness of the symptoms for some women adds to the uncertainty of the disease, not knowing from day to day how their health will be and what impact it will have on their life.

> "I never know how I will feel in the morning, afternoon, or evening. My life is permanently on hold as I never know from one day to another how I will feel." [5]

Conversely, for some women the association with menstruation means that their symptoms are cyclical and predictable, and women with this disease pattern may plan their lives around the 'bad days', ensuring that social events and holidays are, as far as possible, arranged when they are fairly certain they will be relatively pain free. Fluctuations in the disease trajectory can be accommodated within these women's lives. However, even for these women there is less predictability about other symptoms, such as dyspareunia.

When it comes to viewing the future, there is even less certainty. Women know that even if a treatment reduces their pain it may return at any time. This is particularly true of hormonal treatments that mask the pain rather than remove the disease.

The future is often viewed with a mixture of hope and pessimism, hope that a treatment will work, and pessimism knowing that there is no cure and symptoms may recur.

> "I personally don't think I will ever be pain free, and I don't think I will ever get rid of endometriosis." [5]

> "[I feel] rosy but also aware it may come back!! Fingers crossed it doesn't." [5]

The most hopeful women are those who have had some success in treatment, with no setbacks. These tend to be younger women who have had a shorter than average delay in diagnosis. Older women, who may have had many different treatments that relieved the pain for only a short time, have learned that symptoms will recur.

4.5
Impact on Social Life and Relationships

> "I'm blessed with a husband who has stuck through so much and has been to every medical appointment I've ever had. He has held my hand through the internal examinations . . . What would life be like if I didn't have him?" [1]

Social relationships may be the major source of support for women with endometriosis, with partners and family usually providing the most positive support, although, as indicated above, endometriosis can be a factor in the breakdown of relationships. However, some women find that support is time limited, with people being very sympathetic initially, but less so as time goes on, particularly if the woman has had treatment. Friends expect the woman to get better, and will lose patience and drift away when social events are repeatedly cancelled at the last minute.

> "Friends have been really, really good. I think I must be quite lucky with the circle of people that I'm with. They've all been incredibly supportive." [1]

> "[Social activities] just went by the board . . . At the moment, I've got no social life at all." [1]

Even family can find it hard knowing how to react to someone who is in constant or cyclical pain and who does not recover from her illness, and so some women report that endometriosis is a very lonely disease, where no one really knows what they endure.

> "So I've felt it's quite a lonely illness. It's the sort of thing that you're really left with on your own. And it's embarrassing, and it's, you know, shameful, and it's gynecological, and you don't talk about things 'down there'." [2]

Those women with children become concerned about their ability to care for them, and will speak about not being a "proper" mother. They worry about the impact on their children of seeing them in pain, and some women will go to great lengths to hide their pain.

> "All in all I am so fed up with being ill and having to explain to my children that mummy is unwell again today. This is breaking my heart as my children are only 2 and 8 years."

These women may rely on others to do the things for their children that they feel they should do themselves, such as take them to school or play active games. This engenders feelings of guilt, and some women have found this the most difficult part of the disease.

Similarly with work relationships, the quality of the experience is highly dependent on employers' and colleagues' perceptions of and reaction to endometriosis. A positive work experience is characterized by an understanding of endometriosis and how it can lead to sickness absence, and less than optimum performance. For many women, however, employers can be unsympathetic and cause them to feel guilty when taking time off, or to go to work when they are really too ill.

> "I think the doubting is the worst thing. Because it makes you feel like you're a liar, or you are making more of it than perhaps you should." [2]

> "I'd be absolutely fighting to get to work, because I was really worried about having more work, and I had a warning that my sickness rate was unacceptable." [1]

Colleagues can also accuse women of being hypochondriac or of malingering, and resent having to do extra work because of one worker's frequent absence.

> "Somebody said to me 'Look, people were really [annoyed] when you were off because they were having to do your job as well'." [2]

Some women in this situation choose not to disclose their endometriosis to work colleagues for fear of being asked to leave [9]; however, some women also choose to give up work altogether, as the strain of dealing with a reputation as unreliable or work-shy compounds the experience of living with endometriosis.

4.6 Interactions with Health Professionals

As with social relationships, relationships with health professionals may be supportive, or very negative. Most women's initial experience is with a general practitioner (GP)/primary care physician, who may act as gatekeeper to more specialist services and gynecologists. GPs are usually the first point of contact when women decide to seek professional help, and their reaction and response to the presenting symptoms are crucial in determining the experience that will follow. If women are "fobbed off" at this stage, or their symptoms are trivialized or normalized, they will almost certainly experience the delays in diagnosis discussed above.

> "I probably went [to the GP] on and off for quite a while before they sent me. He was always very reluctant to pass me on [to a gynecologist] which has been a lot of wasted time. I'm a bit resentful in that respect." [4]

> "It was like, 'well everyone complains of painful periods' and I was like 'well I can't go to the toilet without it hurting. You know I can't have sex without it hurting, this can't be normal. You're telling me it's normal?'."

Women will often describe their interactions with health professionals as "battles" and feel that they have to struggle for every investigation and treatment.

> "Why do I have to fight to get the treatment I need . . . Why do I have to struggle to get appointments to see people and to be taken seriously?" [2]

Some doctors also perpetuate the myths around endometriosis, that pregnancy will cure it, or that a hysterectomy is the only certain cure. These "solutions" can be particularly distressing to young women, who may then view their options as being limited to being symptom free only by having a child when not mature, or remaining child free.

> "Even my own GP keeps telling me to start a family, that that will cure me. It's knowledge for medical and lay people. I feel that there is just not enough out there." [4]

> "One of the GPs actually told me that period pains didn't exist and it was just women being stupid, so I didn't actually get any painkillers." [4]

Gynecologists who do not have the necessary knowledge and skills to offer the most appropriate diagnostic procedures and therapies can also lead to negative experience and delay, and the most positive experience for women is often when they find a specialist in endometriosis who understands their condition and has expertise in current treatments. However, this is often after many years of false hopes and ineffective treatments.

As with much long-term illness, women become experts in their own condition, and will frequently comment on the lack of knowledge of some health professionals, and, more importantly for them, the lack of willingness to learn about endometriosis or accept information from the patient. Women in this situation feel powerless to use their knowledge to help themselves to achieve better treatment, as they need the cooperation of the medical profession.

> "I went to see a GP, but not the one who had been sympathetic, it was a newly qualified GP. And I felt she was contradicting everything I had read in endometriosis books. So I had no confidence really." [4]

> "He actually said to me 'I don't know this condition at all'." [4]

4.7 Treatments

Although there is no definitive cure for endometriosis, there are many medical and surgical treatments for the disease, as well as symptomatic treatments and alternative therapies.

Drug treatments seem to cause more concern for women than surgery, and even repeated surgery does not seem to raise anxiety about immediate or long-term complications.

> "I've had between eight and ten operations . . . The bulk of them were lasering, zapping the endo, the cysts, which grew back pretty well 18 months to 2 years later." [1]

> "I have had some seven laparoscopies related to endometriosis over the past 10 years and each time, the endometriosis returns after about a year and a half." [5]

Most women view surgical risks as worthwhile in order to alleviate their pain. The exception to this is where there is a possibility that surgery will involve the formation of a stoma.

Many young women are initially given oral contraception, and may only experience symptoms of endometriosis again when this is discontinued. Other medication causes unpleasant side effects and only gives temporary relief at most, and so there is a high noncompletion rate. Some classes of drug that suppress the menstrual cycle induce a temporary menopause, and as fertility is a major issue for a number of women with endometriosis, this is not an acceptable option. Young women in particular find the induction of menopause, with the accompanying symptoms, unacceptable, although some will endure it to be rid of the pain.

"They put me on [nafarelin], which is a hormone nasal spray. I was meant to be on it for 6 months. I had to come off it after 5 months because all my hair – about an inch all round my faceline – had fallen out, and I was really depressed. But I felt ill and my hair was falling out, so you're going to be depressed." [1]

"The danazol initially helped . . . They tried danazol again, and my periods went absolutely haywire. I was probably bleeding more than not. It worked out about 7 days on, 3 days off." [1]

"I don't like the fact that I've had all these chemicals, and am still having chemicals pumped into my body." [5]

4.8 Summary

Living with endometriosis can have a major impact on the lives of women and their families. It can affect every aspect of life, and negatively influence the quality of that life. However, the range of experience is diverse, with some women encountering only minor disruption to their lives, and then only for short periods of time. Over the lifespan this diversity may be apparent within the same women.

There is also diversity in the way that women choose to manage their symptoms. Some will withdraw from normal activities, and say that their life is overwhelmed by endometriosis, while others will try to work through the pain and not give in to it. For some women, preserving fertility is of paramount importance, and however great the pain it is secondary.

Quality of life is affected by the extent of pain, but also by the quality of relationships. Supportive relationships with family, friends, and a partner and sympathetic and knowledgeable treatment by health professionals can help to ameliorate the worst effects of symptoms. Conversely, women who feel that it is a struggle to be taken seriously within the healthcare system, or whose family and friends lose patience with the continued illness, will have an added burden to live with.

By using the words of women with endometriosis it has been possible to capture the reality of living with the disease, and to emphasise the issues that are important to them.

References

1. Denny E. Women's experience of endometriosis. J Adv Nurs 2004;46:641–648
2. Denny E. 'You are one of the unlucky ones': delay in the diagnosis of endometriosis. Diversity in Health and Social Care 2004;1:39–44
3. Denny E, Mann CH. Endometriosis-associated dyspareunia: the impact on women's lives. J Family Plann Reprod Health Care 2007;33:189–193
4. Denny E, Mann CH. Endometriosis and the primary care consultation. Eur J Obstet Gynecol Reprod Biol 2008;139:111–115
5. Denny E. 'I never know from one day to another how I will feel': pain and uncertainty in women with endometriosis. Qual Health Res 2009;19:985–995
6. Cox H, Henderson L, Henderson N, Shi C. Focus group study of endometriosis: Struggle, loss and the medical merry-go-round. Int J Nurs Pract 2003;9:2–9
7. Ballard K, Lowton K, Wright J. What's the delay? A qualitative study of women's experiences of reaching a diagnosis of endometriosis. Fertil Steril 2006;86:1296–1301
8. Manderson L, Warren N, Markovic M. Circuit breaking: pathways of treatment seeking for women with endometriosis in Australia. Qual Health Res 2008;18:522–534
9. Gilmour JA, Huntington A, Wilson HV. The impact of endometriosis on work and social participation. Int J Nurs Pract 2008;14:443–448

Printed in November 2010